Start Hairdressing!

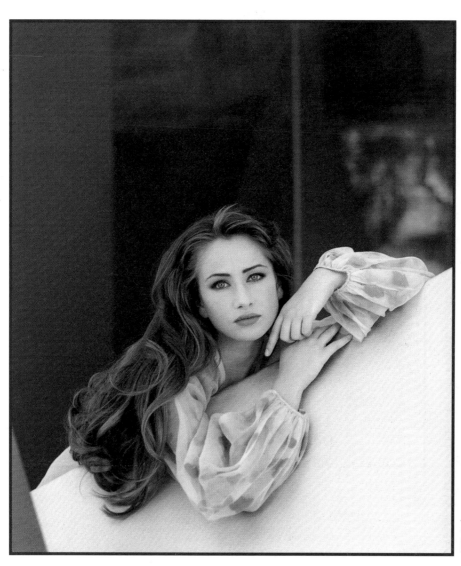

L'Oréal

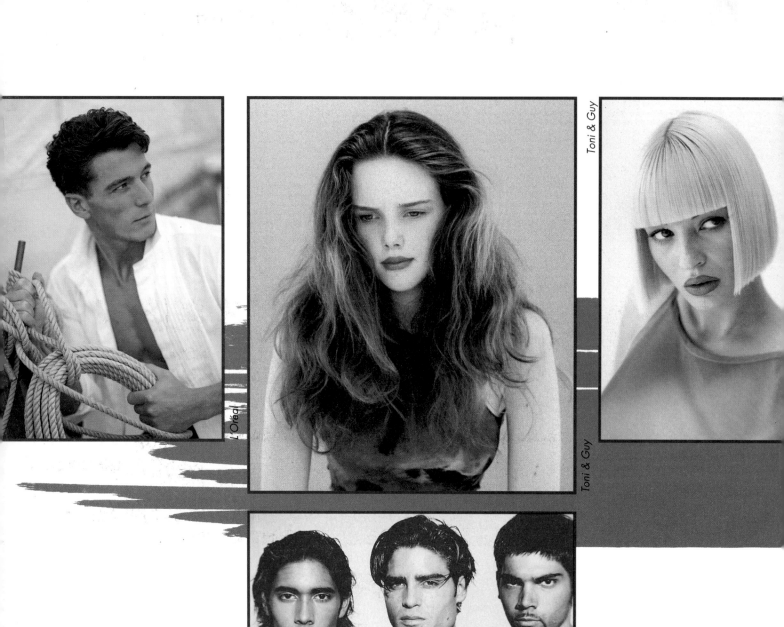

L'Oréal

Toni & Guy

Toni & Guy

Toni & Guy

Start Hairdressing!

The Official Guide to Level 1

by Martin Green and Leo Palladino

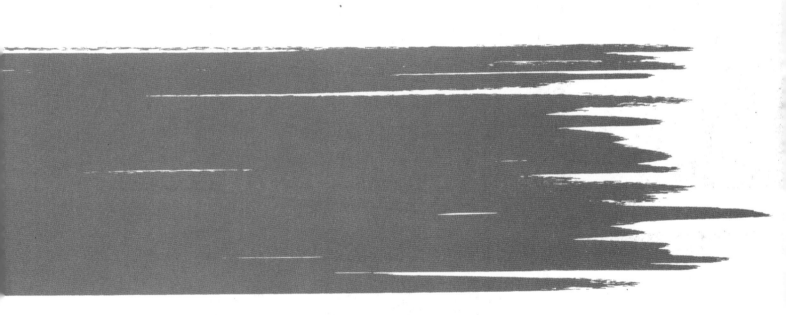

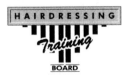

MACMILLAN

Related Macmillan titles

Hairdressing – The Foundations: The Official Guide to Level 2, by Leo Palladino

Professional Hairdressing: The Official Guide to Level 3, by Martin Green, Leo Palladino and Lesley Howson

Patrick Cameron: Dressing Long Hair, by Patrick Cameron and Jacki Wadeson

Beauty Therapy – The Foundations: Level 1 and 2, by Lorraine Nordmann

The Complete Make-Up Artist: Working in Film, Television and Theatre, by Penny Delamar

Manicure, Pedicure and Advanced Nail Techniques, by Elaine Almond

The Nail File, by Leo Palladino and June Hunt

The Science of Cosmetics and *The Beauty Salon and its Equipment*, both by John V. Simmons

The Principles and Practice of Hairdressing, by Leo Palladino

© Martin Green, Leo Palladino and the Hairdressing Training Board 1996

First published 1996 by
MACMILLAN PRESS LTD
Houndmills, Basingstoke, Hampshire RG21 6XS
and London
Companies and representatives throughout the world

ISBN 0–333–65521–4

A catalogue record for this book is available from the British Library.

10	9	8	7	6	5	4	3	2	1
05	04	03	02	01	00	99	98	97	96

Printed in Great Britain by
Scotprint Ltd, Musselburgh

Note about pronouns

Using 'he' or 'she' and 'her' or 'him' throughout the text would become cumbersome in a book such as this. For simplicity, therefore, we have generally used simply 'she' and 'her'.

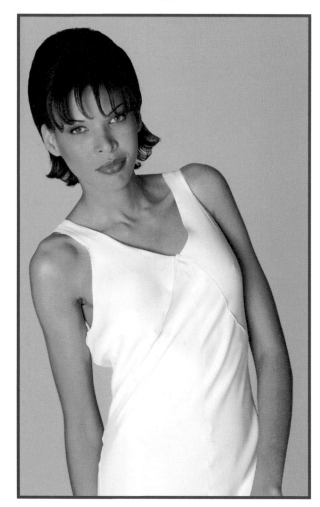

Neville Daniel

Contents

Foreword

Starting work is a real eye-opener! This is the time you learn about work and interaction with other people, mostly older than yourself. One of the most enjoyable and rewarding careers you can go into is hairdressing. Yet hairdressing is not just about hair – it's about people too.

Our standards are high; to be interested in hairdressing is not enough – you need to be determined to meet the standards set by the industry and demanded by clients. To achieve this, your real commitment is one of listening; listen to your supervisors, colleagues and teachers for they are knowledgeable.

When you start your career in hairdressing and you really want to learn, listen to your clients for they are the ones who are the most demanding!

Start Hairdressing today, achieve your qualification and enjoy a fruitful and rewarding career.

Alan Goldsbro
Chief Executive, Hairdressing Training Board

Preface

Start Hairdressing! is your introduction to the exciting and varied world of hairdressing. It aims to illuminate your pathway to success. NVQ/SVQ Level 1, and the needs of associated hairdressing organisations, are fully covered.

This book guides you through some of the practices and techniques involved in hairdressing in a 'helping role'. With experience which you can record in your assessment folder, and regular assessment of your progress, you will gain both the confidence and the skill to approach Level 2.

As your career progresses further you will find that more skills become possible, and what at first appears difficult gradually becomes accomplished and professional. Understanding what you do and how you do it is invaluable in gaining trust and assurance.

With practice and guidance, you will soon become competent. Competence will ensure not only your career satisfaction, but customers who regularly return for all you can offer – the final proof of success.

Martin Green
Leo Palladino

Acknowledgements

The authors and publishers would like to thank the following for providing pictures for the book:

Cheynes Training, City & Guilds of London Institute, Clynol Hair, Comby, Denman, Ellisons, Fire Protection Services, Freeze Frame Photography, Hairdressers Journal International, Hairdressing Training Board, Luster Products Inc., L'Oréal, Mahogany, Neville Daniel, Regis, Smith & Nephew, Toni & Guy, TRESemmé, Wella Great Britain.

The authosr and publishers would also like to thank the following: The Controller of Her Majesty's Stationery Office for Crown copyright material; photographer Steve Whitfield-Almond; Melissa Ashford, Claire Fawlk, Zoe Mitchell, and all the models who were involved in the various technique photographs taken for this book.

Every effort has been made to trace all the copyright holders but if any have been inadvertently overlooked the publishers will be pleased to make the necessary arrangements at the first opportunity.

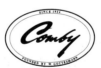

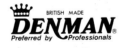

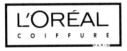

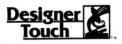

Shampooing and conditioning hair

Shampooing and conditioning are basic hairdressing procedures. They are used to prepare the customer's hair for other processes. Shampooing is the procedure for cleaning both the hair and the scalp: it removes dirt, grease and any other matter that coats them. This cleaning is essential in preparing the hair – any deposits that remain in the hair after shampooing may affect later hairdressing procedures.

Conditioning maintains the hair in a healthy state. It helps to protect and lubricate the hair and keep it pliable. Conditioning also helps to overcome any damage caused by chemical hair processing, enabling the hair to recover its normal elasticity and shine.

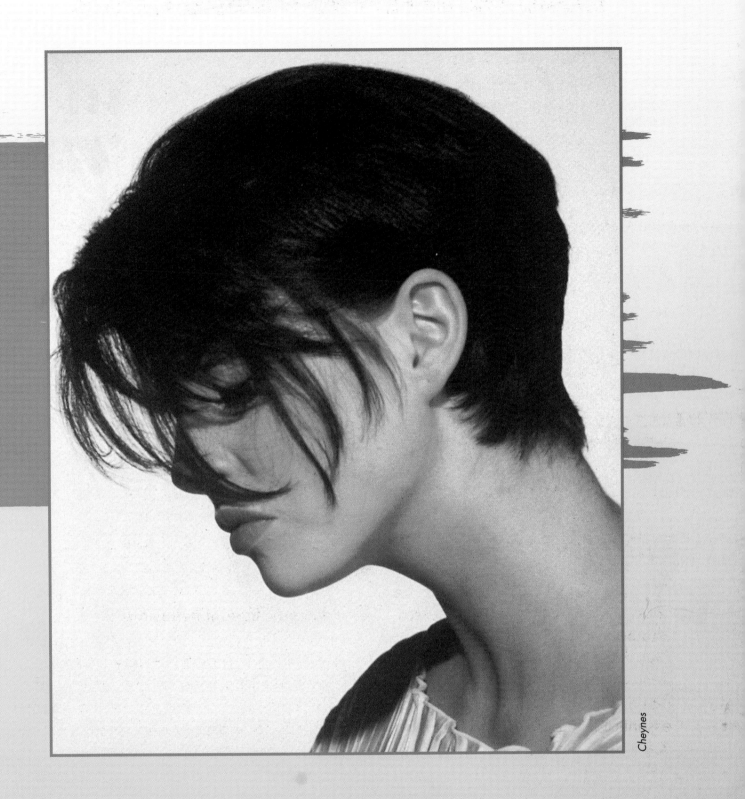

Cheynes

Shampooing

The shampooing process should be soothing, enjoyable and pleasant for your customer. It is one of the first procedures she experiences in the salon, so she is likely to assess the salon's standards from the shampooing. You need to be professional, efficient and caring throughout the process.

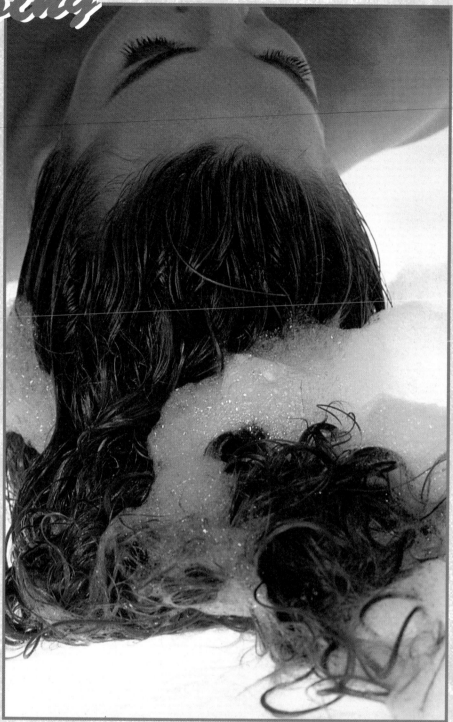

Alex Springer / Camera Press Ltd

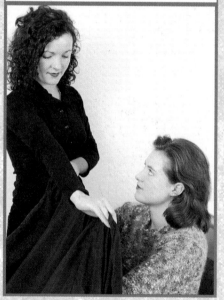

Preparing the customer

1 Preparation **1** Protect your customer's clothes with a gown and towel, placing the towel over her shoulders. Do not tuck tissues or towels into the gown: they might absorb water and make the customer's clothes wet.
2 Reassure your customer – tell her what you are doing, and why.

What's going on?

Your stylist will first:

● discuss with the customer what is required, and determine the hairdressing services to be given

● determine the condition and state of the hair and scalp

● select a suitable shampoo and check the manufacturer's instructions.

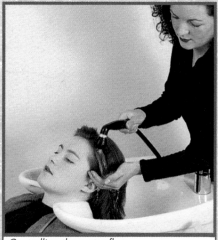

Controlling the water flow

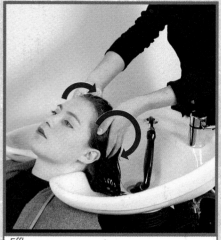

Effleurage movements

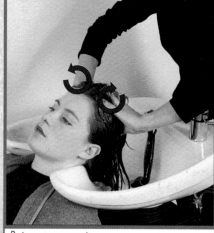

Rotary movements

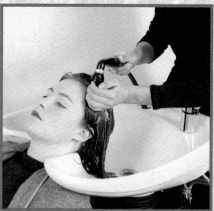

Rinsing

2 Shampooing control

1 Make sure your customer is comfortable at the basin. Check that all of the hair is within the bowl.
2 Run the cold water first, then mix hot water into the cold.
3 Test the water temperature on the back of your hand. After lifting the spray, and before you apply water to your customer's head, check the temperature again. As you work, keep one hand between your customer's head and the water spray – if the temperature changes, you will be aware of it.
4 Check the water pressure and flow. Direct the water flow away from the hairline. Thoroughly wet the hair.

3 Technique

1 Apply the shampoo. First dispense it into the palm of your hand; then spread it evenly, using effleurage hand movements, over the customer's hair and scalp. Position your hands as shown. Cleanse the hair using rotary hand movements.
2 Rinse the hair thoroughly, making sure that the hairline is completely cleared.
3 If the hair and scalp are still dirty, apply more shampoo and repeat the process.
4 Turn off the water. Return the spray head to its place. Wrap the hair with a towel, and reposition your client comfortably.
5 At this stage, apply conditioner if this is required (see page 15).

Tips

▪ Natural hair moisture is lost if the hair is squeaky clean.

▪ To avoid waste, use only a little shampoo, as necessary.

▪ Make sure that your customer is comfortable throughout the shampooing procedure.

▪ When combing, make short rather than long combing movements.

HEALTH AND SAFETY

★ Never apply a shampoo without your stylist's permission.

★ Before and during shampooing, check the water temperature and flow.

★ Always rinse your hands after shampooing. Don't allow shampoo to stay on your hands – it might cause dryness and soreness.

★ Use only clean, unbroken combs, to prevent germs passing from one person to another and to prevent damage to the hair or scalp.

4 Towel-drying, combing and finishing

1 Move your customer from the shampoo area to a clean workstation.

2 Gently squeeze and lightly towel-dry the hair to remove excess moisture. Take care, particularly if the hair is long. Loosen the hair by teasing it apart with your fingers.

3 Comb the hair from the points to the roots. (If you start combing at the roots, the hair will tangle.) Support your customer's head, to avoid discomfort. Comb the hair until it flows freely.

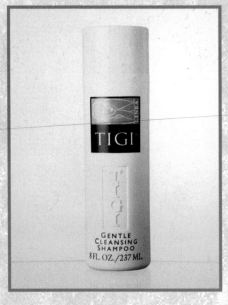

TIGI

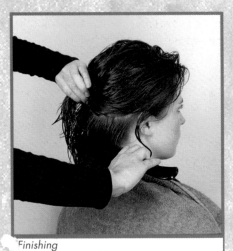

Finishing

4 It is now ready for the hairdressing process to follow. Tell the stylist that you have completed your task.

5 Clean and tidy the shampoo area.

ACTIVITIES

- Examine hair tips – splitting or breakage may indicate that the hair is dry and has been badly treated.

- Take two hairs from the same person. Soak one in water for a minute or two. Stretch the hairs and compare them – hair stretches more when wet than when dry.

- Test hair for elasticity: stretch a dry hair, and note how easily it reverts to its previous length. Healthy hair is very elastic.

- With two or three colleagues, shampoo each other's hair. Notice the different shampooing action used with long and short hair.

Tips

█▄▄▄▄▄▄ If hair is washed daily, one shampoo application is enough. Use two applications only when the hair is very dirty.

█▄▄▄▄▄ Both for care and for safety, assist your customer when moving from the shampoo area.

What does it mean?

The language of hairdressing includes a range of special words and terms with particular meanings. Here are some of them.

hair condition The state of the hair – greasy, dry or normal.
tangle Knotted hair.
disentangle To remove the knots.
hairline The margin between the hair and the skin.
points Free hair ends.
technique A method of doing something.
shampooing The process of cleaning the hair and scalp.
effleurage A light, soothing, stroking massage movement.
rotary In a circular pattern.
professional Trained or skilled to high standards.
stylist A trained, qualified hairdresser.
manufacturer Someone who makes the hairdressing tools and products.
wholesaler Someone who sells large quantities of hairdressing products.

Hairdressers Journal / Comby Matador (Daniel Mollison at John Baxter-Hill, Cobham, Surrey)

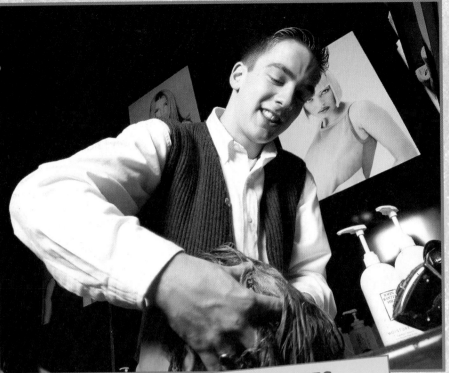

Hair condition

Greasy hair can be difficult to deal with, as it will not easily hold a shape or style for long. The greasiness is due to excessive oil from the scalp. Some shampoos and conditioners are designed specifically for washing greasy hair.

Dry hair can be brittle and liable to break. It may result from a lack of oil in the hair or from chemical treatments or overheating. Dry hair needs careful handling and suitable shampoos and conditioners.

Normal hair is neither too oily nor too dry. It is smooth, shiny, naturally supple and easy to manage. The shampooing and conditioning of this hair type aims to retain its normal, natural condition.

ACTIVITIES

● Find out what types of combs are available, and what the different ones do.

● Find out what types of shampoos your salon uses. Which does it sell for home use?

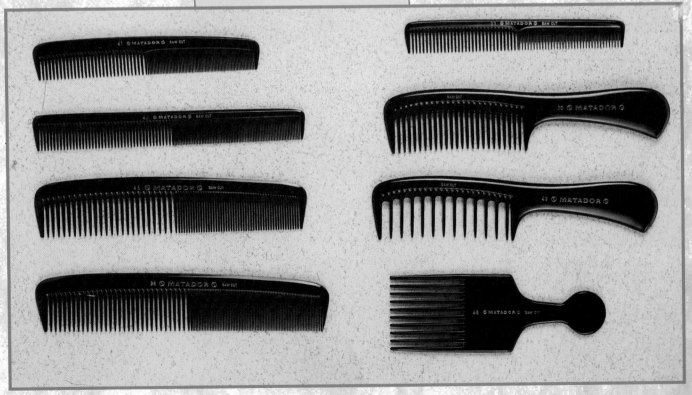

Comby

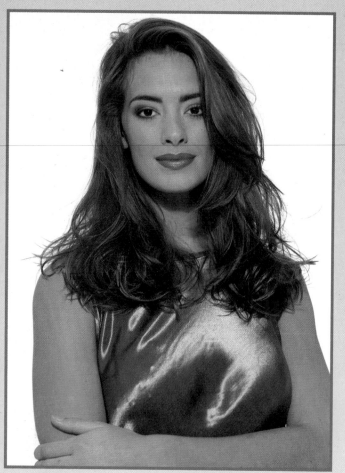

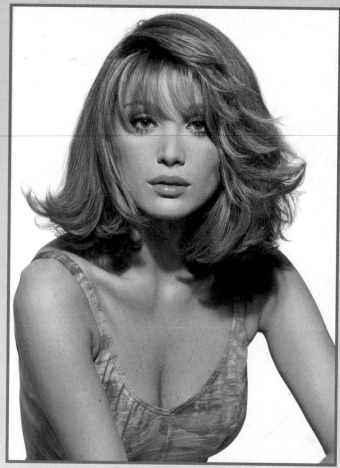

Hair length

Long hair Hair that reaches below the shoulders. Long hair is 'older' and is likely to have had a variety of physical and chemical treatments. It may have a combination of oily roots and dry ends.

Medium hair Hair that reaches just below the nape. Medium hair allows a variety of shapes, if a good condition is maintained.

Short hair Hair kept above the nape. Short hair is 'newer', and may be more resistant to styling and to chemical treatments.

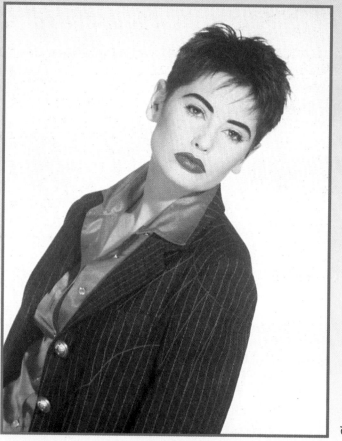

Conditioning

Healthy hair shines, is smooth and pliable, and retains its style and shape. Hair in poor condition looks dull, is inelastic, and is unable to hold a shape. Conditioners and conditioning processes help to maintain healthy hair, and they help to correct hair in poor condition.

What surface conditioners do

Surface conditioners have several functions:
● they add gloss and shine to the hair
● they make the hair easier to manage, and reduce knots and tangles
● they help to balance the effects of chemical treatments, such as perming
● they make the hair more elastic and pliable
● they increase the life of the style and shape
● they counter the effects of dry, brittle, breaking hair and smooth down frizziness
● they moisturise a dry, flaking scalp.

Types of surface conditioner

Surface conditioners come in various forms:
● dressing gels, creams and oils
● reconditioning mousses, creams and lotions
● acid balancers.

What's going on?

Your stylist will select a suitable conditioner.

There are several different types of conditioner. Some coat the outside of the hair and are called *surface conditioners*.

Others penetrate deep into the hair structure and are called *penetrating conditioners*. Some combine the advantages of both types.

At this stage of your training you may be expected to help with the application of surface conditioners.

What does it mean?

Here are some more special terms in the language of hairdressing.

condition The state of the hair.
pliable Bendy; able to be curled and shaped.
brittle Breaks easily.
elastic Stretches and returns to its original length (hair in good condition).
inelastic Stretches, but does not return to its original length (hair in poor condition).
conditioner A product used to improve the state of hair.
surface conditioner A product that coats the hair surface.
penetrating conditioner A product that enters the hair and helps to repair its structure.
special conditioner A conditioner that corrects a specific problem with the hair.
pre-perm A product for use before perming.
post-perm A product for use after perming.

1 Preparation 1 Make sure your customer is comfortable. Protect her clothes with a gown and towels (see page 10).
2 Check that you have selected the right product, according to the manufacturer's instructions.
3 Separate the hair by teasing it apart, so that conditioner can be applied evenly.

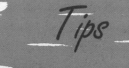

Tips

▮▮▮▮ Before you start any procedure, collect together everything you need – otherwise you'll be running back and forth unnecessarily.

▮▮▮▮ Keep practising – practice will give you confidence.

3 Removal 1 Run the cold water first, then mix hot water into the cold.
2 Test the water temperature on the back of your hand. Check the water pressure and flow. Keep one hand between your customer's head and the water spray.
3 Rinse the conditioner from the hair with warm water, ensuring that all hairlines are cleared.
4 Turn off the water flow. Return the spray head to its place.

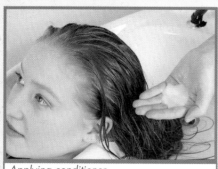
Applying conditioner

2 Application 1 Apply conditioner, first into the palm of your hand: spread it evenly over the hair and scalp. Massage it in using effleurage stroking movements.
2 Comb through the hair so that the conditioner is evenly distributed.

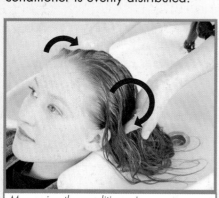
Massaging the conditioner in

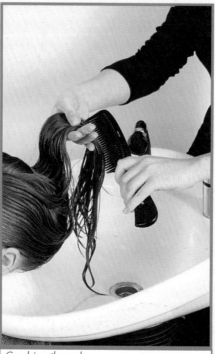
Combing through

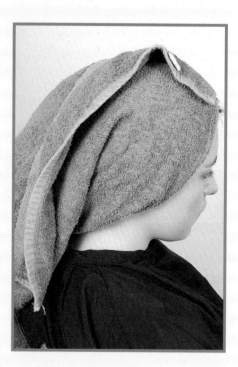

4 Towel-drying, combing and finishing 1 Wrap the hair with a towel. Move your customer to a clean workstation.
2 Gently squeeze and lightly towel-dry the hair to remove excess moisture. Loosen the hair by teasing it apart with your fingers.
3 Comb the hair from the points to the roots.
4 Remove the damp towels and check that your customer is comfortable. Let the stylist know that you have completed your task.
5 Clean and tidy the shampoo area.

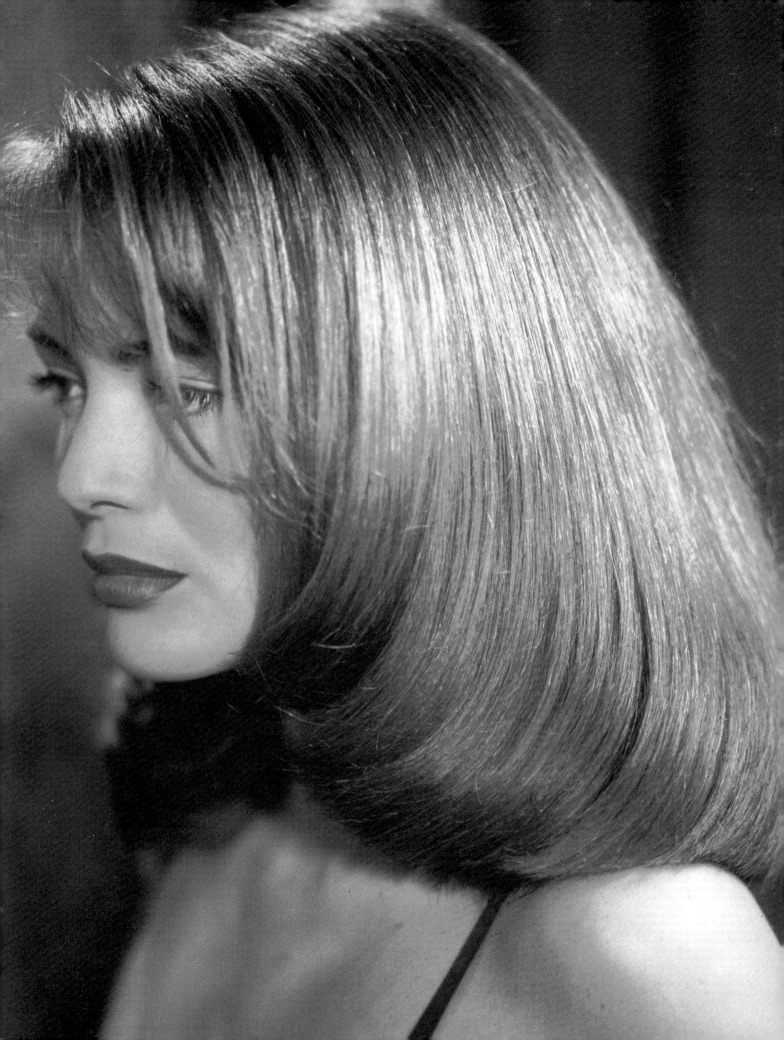

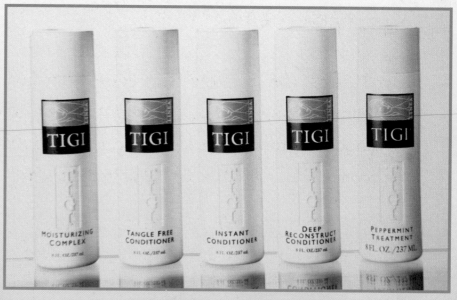

TIGI

▬▭▭▭▭ Professional combs are specially designed for constant use.

▬▭▭▭▭ When you comb hair, start from the points first, and gradually move up the hair length. This is gentler and helps to avoid tangles.

HEALTH AND SAFETY

✳ Always read manufacturers' instructions for use of their products.

✳ Always test water before spraying it onto the customer's hair and scalp.

ACTIVITIES

● Run your fingers through hair and feel it. The smoother, silkier and untangled it is, the better its condition is likely to be.

● Look at hair to see whether it has a natural shine. Dull hair indicates a rough surface and poor condition.

● Visit your local wholesaler and get to know what products are available. Which are recommended for salon use? Which are for home use? Collect and read the manufacturers' instructions.

● On blocks, practise combing, shampooing and conditioning movements.

Assignments

1 List the range of products used in your salon. Collect manufacturers' instructions for these products.

2 Make notes about the process of shampooing and conditioning. Ask yourself questions about them, to understand them better. For example, What is the difference between effleurage and rotary hand movements? When would you shampoo hair more than once? (Keep these notes in your folder.)

More specialised treatments

Penetrating conditioners enter the hair and help to repair its structure. They provide a wide range of treatments:

● before and after chemical treatments (e.g. pre-perm and post-perm)

● to repair damaged, splitting or overprocessed hair (which is very porous)

● to counter dandruff

● to remove excessive greasiness

● to improve hair that is difficult to manage, e.g. fine hair.

Word search

The 10 words listed below are hidden in the diagram.
They have been printed across (backwards or forwards), up or down,
or diagonally, but always in a straight line. You can use the letters in the
diagram more than once. Can you find them all?

SHAMPOOING
GREASY
CONDITIONER
EFFLEURAGE
GOWN
WHOLESALER
COMB
RINSE
BRITTLE
SECTION

C	B	S	E	R	A	W	Q	M	E	G	W	K	L	R
N	O	A	E	G	N	I	O	O	P	M	A	H	S	S
J	S	N	I	P	G	N	U	V	P	E	E	B	R	A
U	X	W	D	A	Q	D	B	U	L	L	D	H	G	W
O	E	E	M	I	P	U	U	T	N	I	L	L	J	H
P	G	F	H	A	T	E	T	C	O	H	J	A	Y	O
L	A	P	E	J	H	I	D	G	I	O	Q	U	F	L
T	R	O	I	R	R	G	O	K	T	U	G	G	N	E
E	U	I	O	B	R	W	S	N	C	S	U	R	U	S
W	E	K	N	N	G	T	E	E	O	W	E	D	A	
W	L	M	S	S	O	I	B	S	S	R	L	A	E	L
H	F	C	S	J	E	E	I	N	P	D	X	S	F	E
A	F	Y	O	L	N	S	H	O	P	I	D	Y	E	R
I	E	E	H	M	Z	R	I	A	O	F	W	F	E	S
D	S	D	Y	F	B	P	E	R	X	D	P	O	R	J

Multiple-choice questions

1 Before any hairdressing process, it is important
a to prepare the customer's hair
b to shampoo the hair
c to curl the hair

2 The word 'shampoo' means
a to press or rub
b to clean
c to condition

3 Which conditioners remain outside the hair?
a penetrating conditioners
b surface conditioners
c foaming conditioners

Drying hair

Styling hair is the process of shaping wet hair while blow-drying it. Usually this follows shampooing. Special care must be taken if blow-drying is to be safely and correctly carried out. You need to follow the stylist's instructions, and you must adopt the correct drying and brushing movements.

Drying the hair involves various techniques which use particular hand movements and applied heat. The aim is not only to remove excess moisture but also to position and shape the hair.

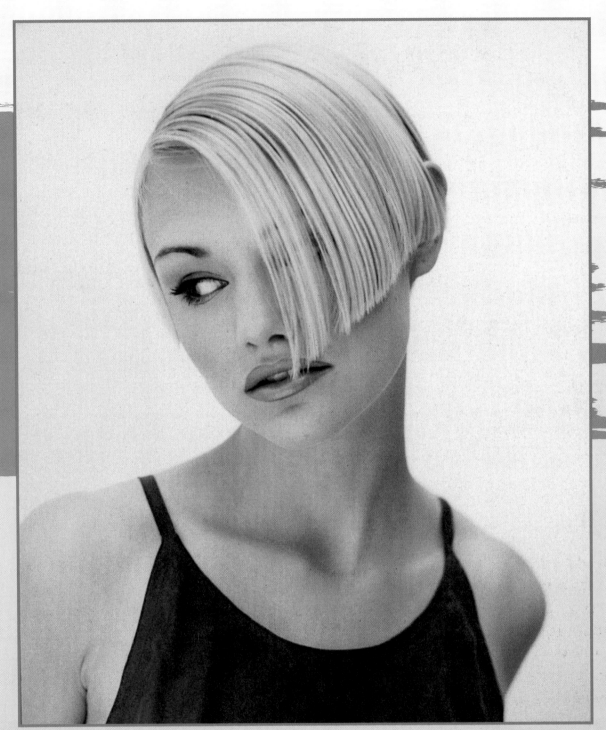

Toni & Guy

Basic principles

Temperature

The switches of a hand-held dryer control the temperature of the air flow. At the beginning of the blow-drying process higher temperatures are used. Cooler air is used to fix the completed style. Your customer should be comfortable throughout the process.

Direction of air flow

The air flow is carefully directed onto small sections of hair which are brushed, combed or pushed by hand into the desired shape. The stream of directed hot air is moved constantly, to avoid burning hair and scalp.

Force of air flow

Initially a greater force of air is used, to remove excess moisture from the wet hair. The hair takes shape later, when it is only slightly damp: at this point greater control and a reduced air flow are required.

What's going on?

● A variety of effects can be produced by drying the hair with hand-held dryers and attachments. The heat softens the hair, which can then be moulded into place. After cooling, it retains its new shape.

● The hair shape is formed and the hair positioned by controlled movements of the brushes and combs.

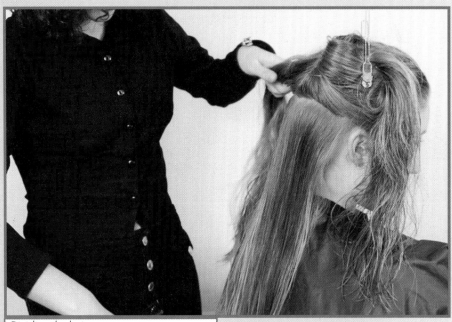

Dividing the hair

Drying long hair

With long hair that is all of one length, the underlying parts of the hair must always be dried first.

1 Sectioning and general drying 1 Divide the hair, using either combs or your fingers, into manageable amounts.

Hair that has yet to be dried should be secured out of the way. (This method is repeated throughout the drying process, allowing careful controlled drying of the hair sections.)

2 Roughly dry all of the hair to remove excess moisture.

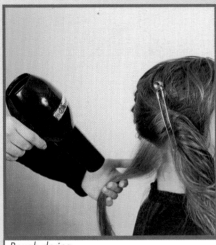

Rough drying

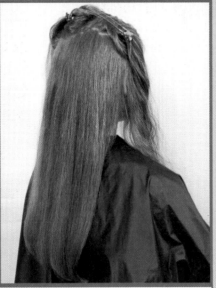

Dried hair before resectioning

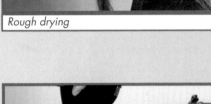

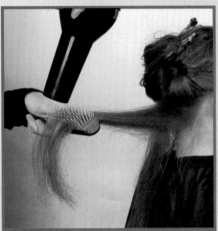

Lifting the hair

3 Before resectioning, ensure that this section is dried. Continue to move the brush away from the head to the hair points, in the same direction as the hairdryer.

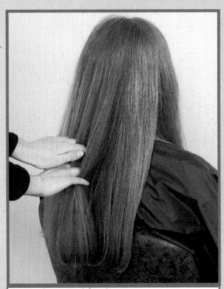

Smoothing and finishing

Tip

▭▭▭▭ Always dry the roots first, before the middle and end parts of the hair section. If you don't do this, the hair won't lie the way you want it to.

Taking care of your customer

Remember:
● excessive drying permanently damages the hair
● insufficient drying causes the shape to be lost
● dry the hair evenly
● don't let the heated air get too hot
● don't let the force of the air flow be too high
● don't let the air inlet of the dryer get blocked
● don't blow hot air too long or too close to the scalp
● don't allow wet hair to fall onto the dried hair
● don't lose control of the hair, blowing it out of shape
● place the dryer safely on the worktop when not in use.

2 Blow-drying   1 You may need to reposition your customer's head to avoid burning her.
2 Working on one hair section, lift the hair so that you can place the brush underneath. Move the brush away from the head towards the points of the hair; follow with the hairdryer, in the other hand, moving in the same direction.

3 Smoothing and finishing   1 Allow the hair to cool. Check that it is completely dry.
2 Brush or comb the hair to even and smooth it into the final shape.
3 When the hair has been dried and shaped it may be dressed with spray or lotion (e.g. hairspray) to help it retain its shape.

Other drying methods

Style and shapes may also be achieved by the following drying methods:

● *natural drying* – just leaving the hair to dry
● *finger drying* – lifting the hair with the fingers while using a hairdryer

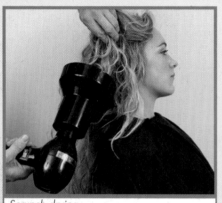

Scrunch drying

● *scrunch drying* – gripping the hair with the hand while using a hairdryer
● drying under a *hood* – this dries the hair quickly, and can be done with or without shaping
● drying under a *heat lamp* – this is slower than using a hood, and is only used when drying without shape
● drying under a *Rollerball* or *Climazone* – machines which produce infra-red heat.

What does it mean?

Here are some more special terms in the language of hairdressing.

blow drying　The method of drying and shaping hair using a hand-held dryer.
hair moulding　Softening and shaping warm hair.
dryer attachments　Pieces fitted onto a hand-held hairdryer – nozzles, diffusers and volumisers.
nozzle　A dryer attachment that directs the air flow.
diffuser　A dryer attachment that reduces the force of the air flow.
volumiser　A dryer attachment that is used to lift the hair.
vent brush　A blow-drying brush that is used to control the hair – its position, volume and direction.

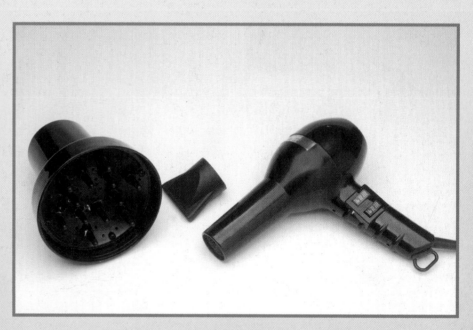

HEALTH AND SAFETY

✶ Never direct heat too close to your customer's scalp. If the heat is too close, you may burn the skin.

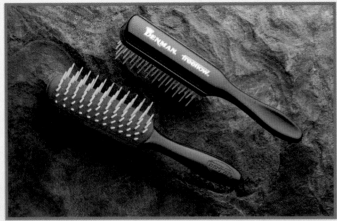

Denman

ACTIVITIES

● Using blocks, practise blow-drying movements.

● Find out what types of brushes are available. What do the different ones do?

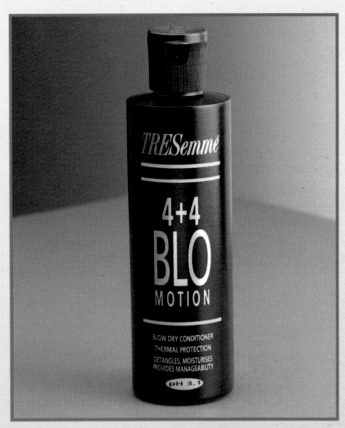

TRESemmé

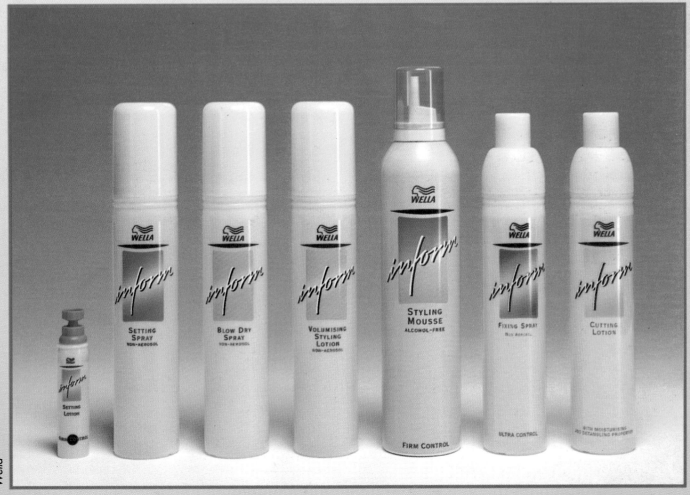

Wella

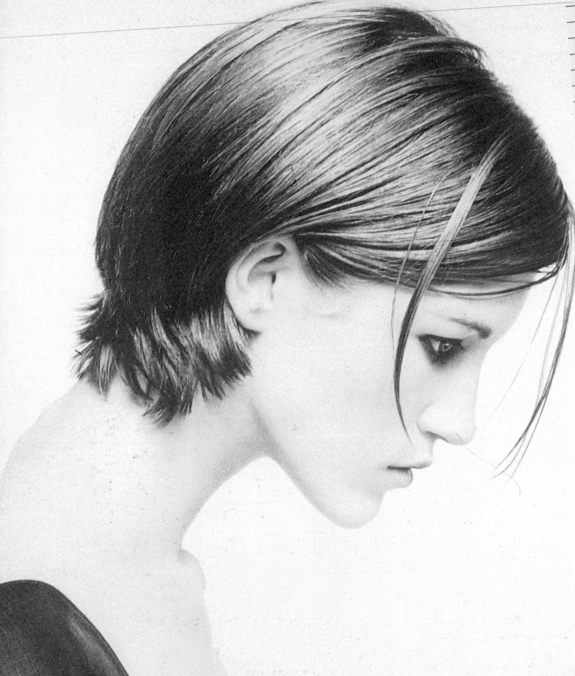

Toni & Guy

Drying hair

1 List the different ways that hair might be damaged by applied heat.

2 Other than blow-drying, what other methods are there for drying hair? Make notes on these, and add them to your folder.

Word search

The 10 words listed below are hidden in the diagram.

They have been printed across (backwards or forwards), up or down, or diagonally, but always in a straight line. You can use the letters in the diagram more than once. Can you find them all?

BLOW-DRYING
DIFFUSER
VENTBRUSH
HEAT
NOZZLE
MOULDING
HAIRSPRAY
SECTION
HAIRDRYER
TEMPERATURE

F	O	A	U	L	C	S	V	H	Y	W	V	R	L	S
S	H	A	I	R	D	R	Y	E	R	K	E	W	W	T
B	Y	F	M	A	E	S	W	E	J	S	N	E	O	E
M	T	W	G	G	A	K	K	Z	U	Y	T	N	D	M
T	S	L	X	T	G	H	O	F	G	F	B	D	D	P
E	A	O	F	N	E	A	F	F	T	S	R	S	M	E
C	Y	E	W	L	R	I	F	I	T	A	U	K	Z	R
I	B	L	O	W	D	R	Y	I	N	G	S	Q	U	A
C	S	Z	A	N	M	S	M	Z	D	C	H	E	A	T
T	I	Z	P	M	P	E	Z	Y	H	Z	Z	L	U
O	S	O	I	W	G	R	L	C	W	T	S	S	A	R
A	S	N	S	M	D	A	Y	O	T	H	Y	K	M	E
F	F	A	W	L	U	Y	J	L	T	I	T	H	A	I
I	S	B	L	Y	O	P	S	O	B	D	O	O	L	L
Y	A	O	K	D	X	M	O	U	L	D	I	N	G	S

Multiple-choice questions

1 What would happen if you held a hand-dryer too close to the client's hair while blow drying?
  a you would burn your hand
  b the heat would burn and damage the hair
  c the heat would bleach the hair

2 For safety, which should you keep checking?
  a the comb
  b the air temperature
  c the brush

3 Which should be dried first?
  a the ends
  b the middle parts
  c the roots

Helping with chemical treatments

Perming and colouring are important chemical processes used in hairdressing. In this chapter we will be looking at the procedures for neutralising perms, adding temporary colourants, and removing colourants from the hair.

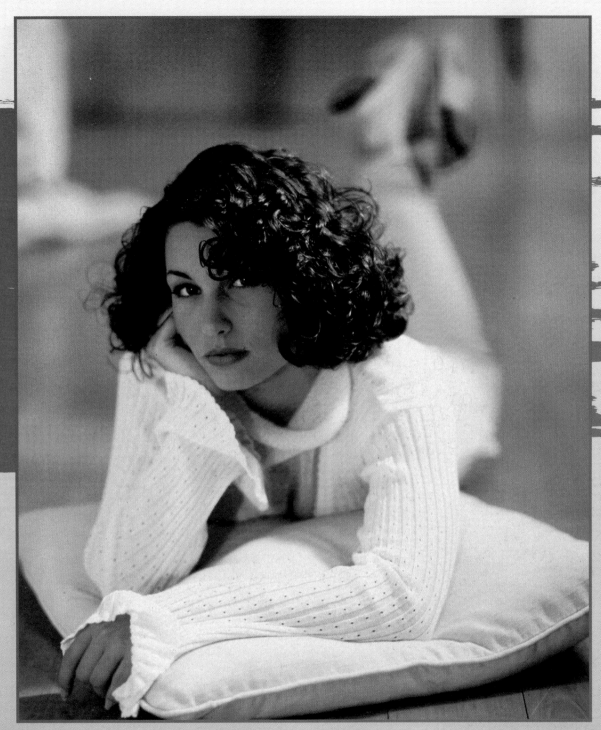

Wella

Perm neutralising

Perm neutralising is the chemical process applied to the hair after it has been permanently curled or waved. Neutralising balances out the hair structure, leaving it in a normal state.

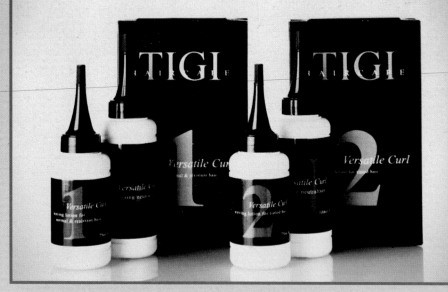

What's going on?

● During perming the hair is softened, stretched and moulded into a waved shape. The hair is then rinsed with water, to dilute the perm and stop the perm action. Neutralising fixes the waved shape into its new position.

● Each perm solution has its own neutraliser, which must be used if the perm is to be effective. The person responsible for the perm will follow the manufacturer's instructions throughout the process.

Equipment and materials

● Clean, fresh, dry towels.
● Neutralising applicators – sponges, brushes, bottles or whatever is required.
● Towels or tissues – to protect the customer's eyes and face.
● The correct neutraliser.

● Cottonwool.
● A measuring jug.
● A timer.
● Gloves – to protect your hands.

Tips

 Always use clean curlers. (Dirty curlers could cause patchy effects.)

 Wash and dry curlers when you've finished with them, so that they are ready for the next customer.

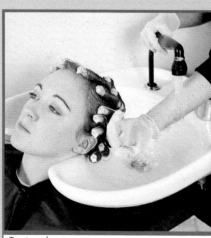

Testing the water temperature

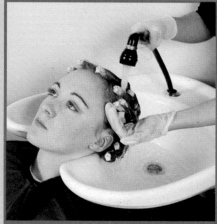

First rinsing

1 First rinse It is important not to loosen the curlers, as this would affect the perm result. If you *do* accidentally loosen any, tell your supervisor immediately.

1 Protect your customer's clothes (see page 10).
2 Test the water temperature.
3 Using a gentle flow of warm water, rinse the hair thoroughly until

all perm lotion has been removed. Do not disturb the wound curlers, but make sure that each curler is thoroughly rinsed. Rinse for as long as necessary, according to the manufacturer's instructions.
4 Carefully blot the hair using a clean towel. To remove surplus moisture, it may be necessary to blot each curler individually with cotton wool.

What does it mean?

Here are some more special terms in the language of hairdressing:

perming The chemical process of making hair wavy.
neutralising The final chemical process when perming hair.
neutraliser A chemical used to stop perm action and to fix the curl.
relaxed hair Hair that has been chemically straightened.
end paper A tissue or wrap, used during winding to secure hair points.
manufacturers The makers of hairdressing or other products.

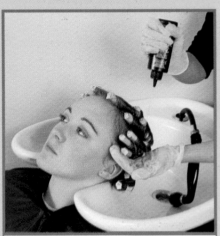
Applying neutraliser

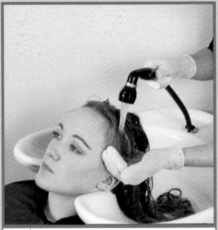
Final rinsing

Neutralising chemically relaxed hair

When neutralising chemically relaxed hair, always follow specific manufacturers' instructions.

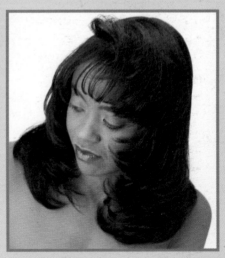
Luster

2 First application
1 Protect your hands.
2 Apply the prepared neutraliser to each and every wound curler, according to the manufacturer's instructions. Wound hair not covered with neutraliser is likely to become weak or straight. Ensure that the neutraliser is well worked in.
3 Leave the neutraliser for the correct time. Always use a timer for accurate processing.

3 Second application
1 Unwind the curlers carefully. Remove any end papers.
2 Carefully apply neutraliser to the unwound hair, making sure that the hair is fully covered. Leave to process according to the manufacturer's instructions.

4 Final rinsing 1 Rinse the hair thoroughly for the second time.
2 Condition the hair (see page 15) if this is recommended by the manufacturer of the neutraliser.
3 Towel-dry the hair to remove excess moisture.

HEALTH AND SAFETY

★ Always protect your hands with gloves or barrier cream.

★ To get good results, apply treatments accurately and check the timing.

★ Check that you are using the right neutraliser! (If you use the wrong one, the perming action might continue, and the hair would become dry and broken.)

★ Always unwind curlers right to the end, to avoid tugging.

★ If you spill neutraliser onto clothes, tell your supervisor immediately.

Adding temporary colour

Adding temporary colour to the hair produces a variety of shades, which can easily be removed. A variety of temporary colour products are available, as setting lotions and creams, mousses and gels, and colour-enhancing shampoos.

Tip

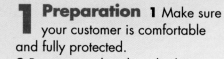 Other types of temporary colour products available include coloured sprays and lacquers, crayons, paints, glitterdust and powders. These are used for special effects.

What's going on?

Adding temporary colour to the hair involves coating the hair with artificial colour. This does not penetrate into the hair structure, but remains firmly attached to the surface until it is washed off. Your stylist will choose a colouring product suited to the particular customer.

1 Preparation 1 Make sure your customer is comfortable and fully protected.
2 Protect your hands with gloves.

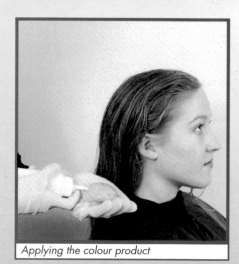
Applying the colour product

2 Application 1 Apply the colour product according to the manufacturer's instructions. Depending on the colour product used, application may be made with a brush, a sponge, an applicator, or direct from the container.

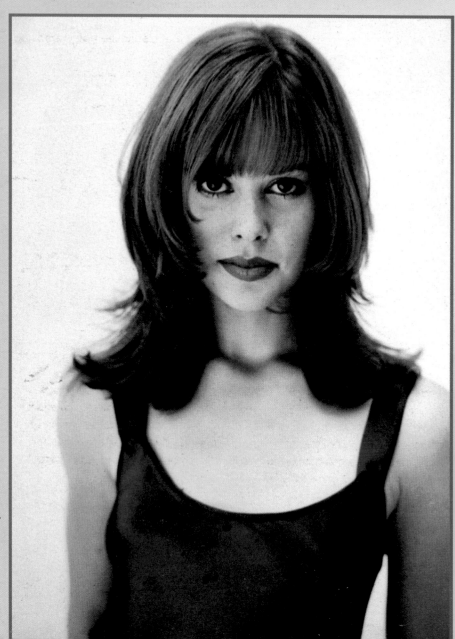

Toni & Guy

Tip

For some temporary colouring products the hair has to be sectioned before application, to ensure even coverage.

What does it mean?

Here are some more special terms in the language of hairdressing.

hair colouring The process of adding artificial colour to hair.

colourant Any type of colouring product used on hair.

surface-coating colour A temporary colourant.

temporary colouring A hair colouring that is washed away by shampooing.

colour shampoo A colouring product that cleans the hair, removing old colour and adding new at the same time.

virgin hair Hair that has not previously been coloured or processed.

processed hair Hair that has been permed or coloured.

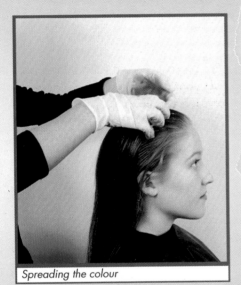

Spreading the colour

2 Spread the colour through the hair. Comb through the hair to distribute the colour evenly.

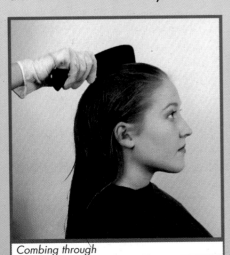

Combing through

Advantages of temporary colouring

Temporary colouring hair has several advantages compared with permanent colouring.

● Most types of temporary colouring do not require mixing.

● The colourants coat the hair surface – they do not get into the hair structure, and can easily be removed by shampooing.

● Soft tones can be added to grey, white or normal hair.

● Fashion effects can be created with hair that has been lightened.

● The colour effects are not long-lasting. This is a safe way for the customer to try out colour without committing herself.

Removing colour

Whereas *temporary colour* only coats the surface of the hair, *semi-permanents* penetrate more deeply and last longer. *Permanents* and *lighteners* also have long-lasting effects.

To remove them, semi-permanents are usually rinsed from the hair. Some may need to be shampooed from the hair.

Permanent colours, lighteners and bleaches, however, may require *emulsifying* – a process of combining or mixing them with water – before rinsing or shampooing the hair in the usual way.

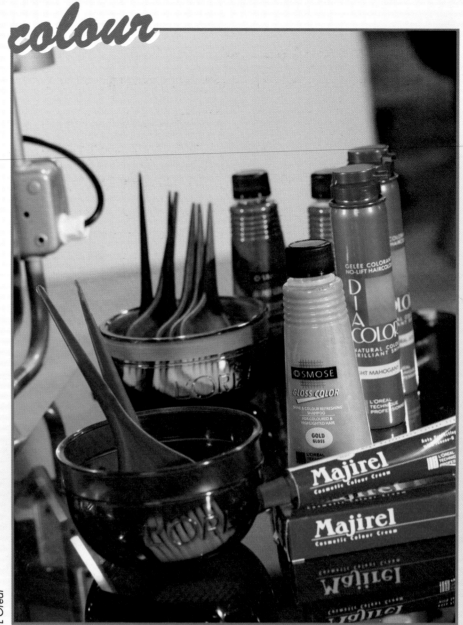

L'Oréal

What's going on?

● There are many ways in which hair can be coloured. Apart from 'full head' application or 'root' application, stylists can also create a variety of effects through *highlighting*, *lowlighting* and other partial-colouring techniques. These make use of caps, foils, wraps, and the like.

● Your stylist will apply the appropriate colouring product and will ask you to remove the surplus colour after processing.

1 Removing surplus colour after using a cap 1 Rinse the hair, to remove surplus colouring product (typically semi-permanent colour or bleach).
2 Apply conditioner, which softens the hair and enables the cap to come off more easily.
3 Remove the cap: lift the rim all the way round, and gently pull the cap away from the head. Be careful not to tangle the hair and cause your customer discomfort.
4 Shampoo the hair in the usual way.

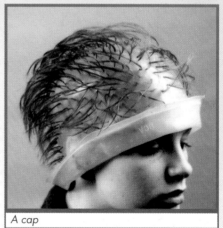

A cap

What does it mean?

Here are some more special terms in the language of hairdressing:

semi-permanent colouring A hair colouring that lasts through several shampoos.

permanent colouring A hair colouring that remains until the hair is cut or grown out.

lightener A bleach or 'lift' colourant, used to make the hair lighter in colour.

bleach A chemical that removes natural hair colour.

highlighting The process of shading or tinting parts of the hair (using tint or bleach) to enhance the style.

lowlighting The process of shading or tinting parts of the hair with subtle shades to enhance the style.

emulsification The process of combining colourants with water.

cap A cap of rubber or plastic, with evenly placed holes through which strands or strips of hair can be pulled for colouring.

wraps Packets used to enclose the parts or strips of hair to be coloured.

foils Packets used to enclose the parts of hair to be bleached or tinted.

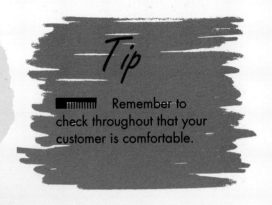

Tip

Remember to check throughout that your customer is comfortable.

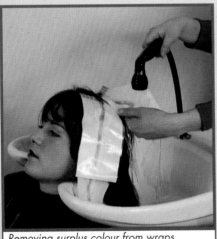

Removing surplus colour from wraps

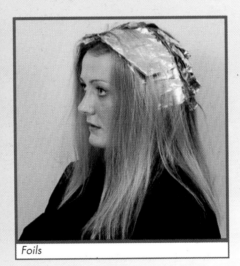

Foils

ACTIVITY

Visit your local wholesaler. Look at the range of temporary colouring products available. Make notes of the differences between them, and collect information leaflets.

2 Removing surplus colour from hair in packets, foils or wraps, when more than one colour is being used

1 Work upwards from the nape of the head to the top and front area. Remove each packet or parcel individually. Rinse this one thoroughly before moving onto the next – insufficient rinsing at this stage will allow the colours to merge during the shampoo process.

2 Shampoo the hair in the usual way.

HEALTH AND SAFETY

★ Check for skin staining. If the skin is stained, clean it as soon as possible. A special stain remover may be necessary – check with your stylist first.

★ When removing colourants from the hair, make sure they don't run over the customer or her clothes.

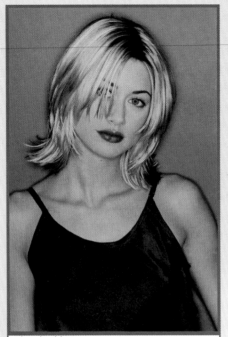

Toni & Guy

Bleached hair

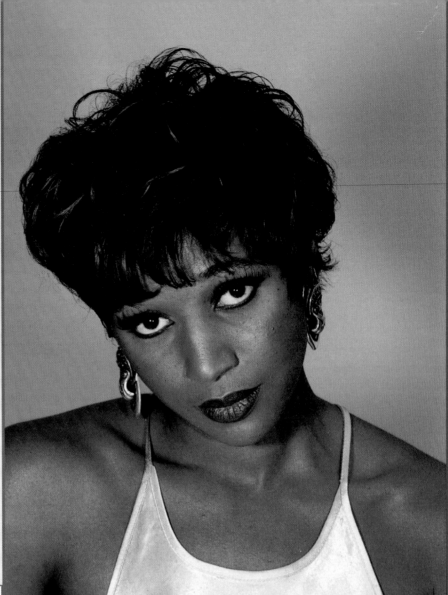

Luster

Coloured hair

Assignments

Neutralising

1 What part does neutralising play in the process of perming hair?

2 What are the possible problems if neutralising is carried out incorrectly?

3 Why is timing so important?

4 Why is it important to wear protective clothing when handling chemical products?

Assignments

Adding temporary colour

1 Describe the various ways of applying temporary hair colour. Illustrate these techniques with sketches. Mention the possible effects of temporary colour on hair. (Keep your notes to add to your folder.)

2 Why is it important to follow instructions?

Assignment

Removing colour

1 Describe the ways in which full head colour and foil highlights should be removed. Include illustrations. (Add these notes to your folder.)

Word search

The 10 words listed below are hidden in the diagram.

They have been printed across (backwards or forwards), up or down, or diagonally, but always in a straight line. You can use the letters in the diagram more than once. Can you find them all?

GLOVES
NEUTRALISER
PERMING
CURLERS
TEMPORARY
VIRGIN
PERMANENT
COLOURANT
BLEACH
INSTRUCTIONS

A	W	F	H	S	V	I	R	G	I	N	T	A	I	C
J	X	U	F	I	O	W	C	W	L	Y	T	Y	C	E
E	H	C	A	E	L	B	D	S	M	O	I	S	T	Y
E	F	N	S	L	S	C	I	R	A	D	V	I	R	M
R	S	L	R	N	C	L	N	E	X	A	M	E	E	B
K	Y	P	T	A	O	B	T	L	N	T	M	S	S	S
L	R	E	W	L	L	I	T	R	I	G	H	S	I	P
P	A	T	E	I	O	S	T	U	T	N	A	R	L	S
U	R	I	B	F	U	T	M	C	F	I	B	S	A	X
Q	O	M	L	L	R	T	H	R	U	M	T	A	R	O
W	P	E	R	M	A	N	E	N	T	R	S	Y	T	B
E	M	N	A	S	N	E	T	X	T	E	T	I	U	L
Y	E	J	L	A	T	M	Y	O	D	P	S	S	E	P
B	T	L	D	Y	L	L	I	R	T	O	I	F	N	C
N	O	S	E	S	Z	A	A	U	L	O	S	A	O	I

Multiple-choice questions

1 What is 'neutralising'?
a curling hair
b perming hair
c balancing hair structure

2 Which colour lasts the longest?
a temporary colour
b permanent colour
c semi-permanent colour

3 Which of the following is a method of removing colour?
a neutralising
b oxidising
c emulsifying

Helping in reception

*B*efore anyone touches her hair, the customer has to be received into the salon. Reception is the point at which she begins her relationship with the salon's staff.

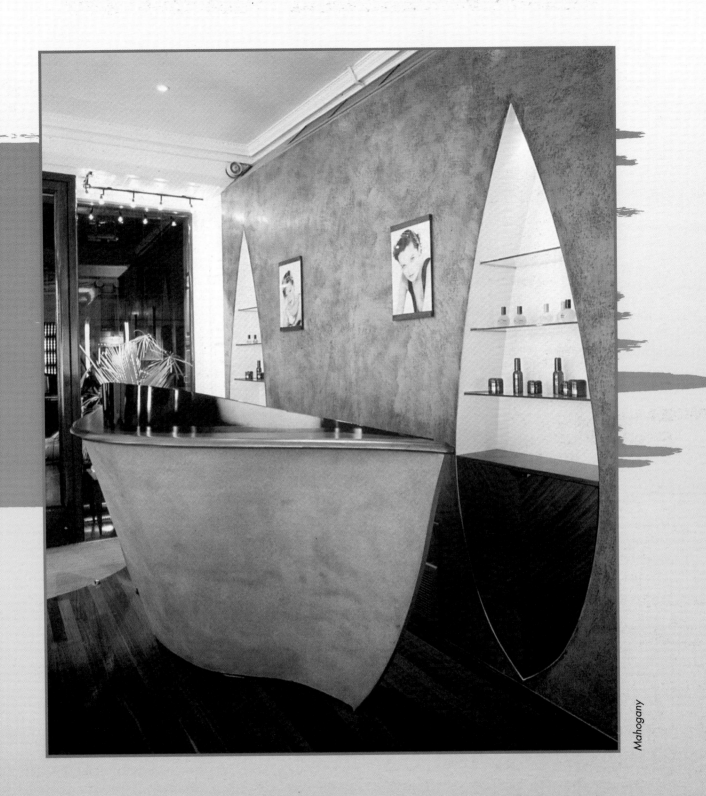

Mahogany

Reception

Reception is an *area* within the salon; it is also the *process* of greeting and welcoming customers, sales representatives and other visitors. At reception you deal with people and attend to their needs.

To be able to attend to customers and enquiries, you need to be prepared:
● always be clean and tidy
● be sure that you understand the salon's appointment system.

While you are talking with a customer:
● look after them
● be pleasant and polite
● listen carefully
● explain and discuss the salon's services as necessary.

When customers have come for hairdressing services:
● assure them of the safety of their belongings.

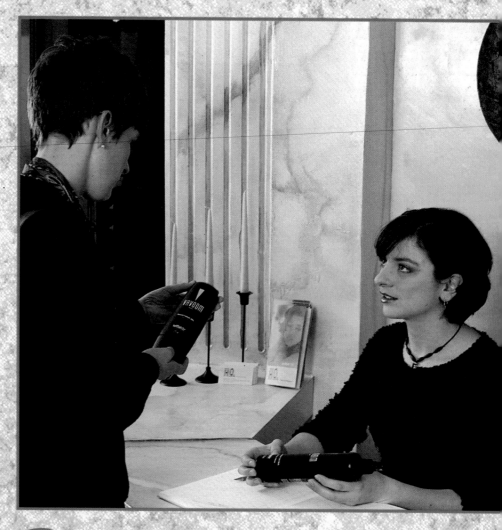

What's going on?

The reception area is the hub of the salon. It is where customers are first met and welcomed; where appointments are made, by telephone and in person; and where products are sold. All till transactions are carried out here.

Receiving visitors

Customers have a number of questions concerning the suitability and cost of the services, goods or products on sale, how long services take, and whether staff are qualified or not. Urgent matters that you cannot handle should be referred to your supervisor immediately.

Tradespeople also may call, to deliver stock, to service equipment or to clean the windows. You need to deal with them courteously and efficiently, so that customers are not inconvenienced and procedures are not delayed.

While you are at the salon, you are at work. Try to discourage friends and relatives from contacting you during business hours, either in person or by telephone.

1 Receiving customers for appointments

1 Meet and greet the customer, and smile. Ask 'How may I help you?'
2 Listen carefully. Show that you have understood the information given.
3 Confirm the appointment.
4 Show the customer where to sit, and offer her magazines or a drink.
5 Inform the relevant staff member as soon as possible that the customer has arrived.

● Remember – if there is anything that you cannot deal with yourself, refer it to your supervisor immediately. Failure to do this could result in customer dissatisfaction and possible loss of business.

2 Taking messages

1 Always listen carefully, and be helpful and polite in your reply.

2 Write down the message received. The message must be readable, accurate, and understandable.

3 Make sure you pass the message to the person intended. (All messages should be in confidence.) Mark the message book to indicate that this has been done.

4 If the person for whom the message is intended is not available, tell others in the salon that there is a message for that person. Check later that the message has been received.

5 If a message requires a reply, or if you have promised to call back, make sure that this is done.

TELEPHONE MESSAGE

To Suzie   Date 15/10

From Ms L White   Time 10.45

Number 23456   Taken by Jean

Please could you call Ms White regarding her appointment tomorrow.

Dealing with people

Hairdressing is a 'people' business. It relies on the employers and employees, the owners of the salons and their staff, all working together. All concerned aim to meet customers' requirements and to ensure each customer's safety and comfort throughout her visit to the salon.

Dealing with people requires good communication. This involves first listening carefully, and then interpreting what is said in order to understand what the customer wants. You can then judge whether the salon is able to satisfy these wants.

Different kinds of communication

We communicate in different ways. We use words, of course (verbal communication) in the salon, but we also use expressions and actions (non-verbal communication).

Talking with your colleagues and customers will be the usual kind of verbal communication in the salon, but you'll also need to write occasionally. The English language is spoken with a rich variety of accents and sometimes uses dialect words: you need to be sure that you understand the other person, and that she can understand you.

Non-verbal communication includes all sorts of things – the way you stand, move, look or act, even without saying anything, can send a variety of messages without you realising it! You can use non-verbal signals positively, making gestures that support what you are saying and that make it easier to understand, and smiling and moving gently. These will attract a favourable response. But beware of giving negative non-verbal signals, such as looking bored, irritable or impatient.

Keep it confidential

In the salon you often hear things that are private and personal: they must not be discussed or repeated. You do not want to cause your customer embarrassment. Information confidential to your customer should be respected at all times.

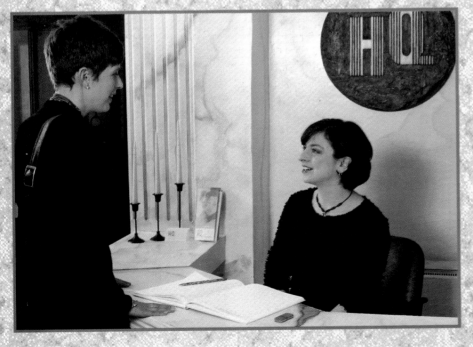

Answering the telephone

The telephone is a vital item in the running of the salon and in making appointments. Telephone conversations must be carefully handled so that communication is effective, and so that you leave the customer with a good impression.

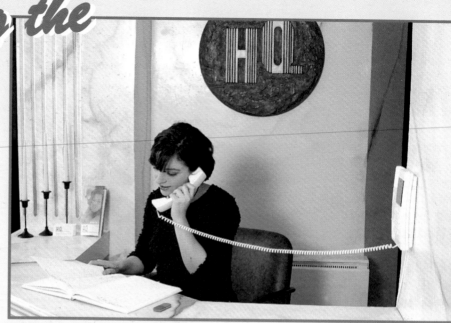

Answering the telephone

1 Answer the telephone promptly, ideally between two and eight rings.
2 Speaking directly and clearly into the telephone, state the salon's name and your own name, and ask how you can help the caller. 'Good morning, Headquarters; this is Alex speaking. How may I help you?'
3 Listen carefully to what the caller says, and record the caller's name. If there is a message, write it down. If the caller is making an appointment, record details in the appointment book.
4 Repeat the details to the caller to confirm them.
5 Thank the caller for ringing, and say goodbye.

Making appointments

When a customer calls to make an appointment, record her name and the service she wants. If the caller is a new customer she may be asked to come in for an initial consultation before making an appointment for services. Check with your supervisor if necessary.

For the efficient running of the salon, you must make appointments accurately and fit in as many as possible. You must allow enough time for stylists to do their work, but not leave too long so that they have nothing to do. For this reason, you need to know exactly how much time your salon allows for each service. If the customer requests a particular stylist, be sure to enter the customer's name in the correct column. Take the customer's telephone number, in case the stylist falls ill or is unable for some other reason to keep the appointment.

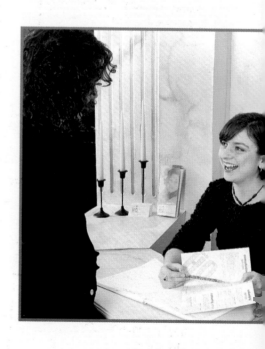

Stylist	Kate	Charlotte	Sally	Sarah	David	Tony		
8:30	Jackson	Lisa			Osborn			
8:45	Wedding B/D	Wedding Put up	Beatrice	Beatrice	Wedding B/D			
9:00	Smith	Cane	Extensions	Extensions	Burtwell	Morley		
9:15	CBD	P/W	Top Only	Top Only	B/D	Meche HL		
9:30	Johnstone	Jacobs			Thomas	Long Hair		
9:45	P/W	Col			Few Meche			
10:00	Williams	Meek D/C			Garner			
10:15	CBD	Cooper D/C			CBD			
10:30	Russell D/C	Cane			Meche			
10:45	Russell D/C	P/W CBD			CBD	Simmons		
11:00	Johnstone	Jacobs			Jorden	CBD		
11:15	P/W CBD	Col CBD			Semi Col	Meche HL		
11:30	Davis	Webster			Godwin D/C	CBD		
11:45	B/D	CBD	Gibbon	Grace	Semi Col	Jackson D/C		
12:00	LUNCH	Passee	CBD	CBD	CBD	LUNCH		
12:15		CBD	Jouhet D/C		Medwell			
12:30		Waldren			B/D			
12:45		CBD	LUNCH	LUNCH	Casey D/C			
1:00	Watts					Beezer		
1:15	Meche HL					HL		
1:30		LUNCH	Gladstone	Crane	LUNCH	Jenkins		
1:45			Spiral P/W	Straightener		Top P/W		
2:00		Peters	(Long hair)	Corker	Cook	Jarvis		
2:15	John	Semi Col		Col	CBD	CBD		
2:30	CBD	Bore D/C	Payne	Straightener	+ Plait	Beezer		
2:45	Tyler D/C	Semi Col	S/set	CBD	Masters	HL CBD		
3:00	Watts	CBD	Selwyn D/C	Corker	P/W	Jenkins		
3:15	Meche CBD	Baker	S/set +Brush	Col CBD	Tozer	P/W CBD		
3:30	Richmond	P/W	Gladstone	Jennings	HL	Gribble		
3:45	CBD	Rickets	P/W CBD	CBD	Smith	Put up		
4:00	Hobbs	CBD	Toby	Osborn	CBD			
4:15	Plait	Griffiths	Put up	CBD	Masters	Salter		
4:30	Simons	BID		Adams	P/W CBD	CBD		
4:45	CBD	Baker	Curtis	CBD	Tozer	Sadler D/C		
5:00	Robins	P/W CBD	CBD	Stevens	HL CBD	Collins		
5:15	CBD			CBD		CBD		
5:30								
5:45								

Date: Saturday 21 September

high Hair

Some points to remember

- Longer services, such as perming, are usually best booked for the early morning or early afternoon so that other services may be fitted in around them.
- A stylist working without help will need more time than one working with help.
- Never fit in an extra appointment without first checking with the stylist concerned.
- Always write clearly so that others can see what you have written, and write in pencil so that the appointment can be erased if it is cancelled or changed.

The appointments diary

The hours of the day are usually printed along the left-hand side of the appointment page, divided into fifteen-minute intervals.

Services are recorded in an abbreviated form. All those who use the appointment page must be familiar with the abbreviations. Here are some common abbreviations:

Service	Abbreviation
Cut and blow dry	C B/D
Blow dry	B/D
Shampoo and set	S/S
Cut, shampoo and set	C S/S
Permanent wave	P/W
Tint	T
Highlights	H/L
Lowlights	L/L

What's going on?

- Each salon has its own system for making appointments. This involves allocating the time that is to be given to each client, depending on the services requested.

- Making appointments is a two-way communication process, whether on the telephone or face to face. You need to give and receive information and record the relevant details.

Appointment cards

An appointment card may be offered to the customer, to confirm the appointment. The card should record the service, the date, the day and the time. The stylist's name may also be included.

Your next appointment	
Date......................................	Time...........................
Date......................................	Time...........................
Date......................................	Time...........................
Date......................................	Time...........................
Date......................................	Time...........................
Date......................................	Time...........................
	Thank you

Tips

▮▦▦▦ Before asking a telephone caller to 'hold on', make sure first that she is willing to wait.

▮▦▦▦ Try always to offer a customer a choice of appointment times.

What does it mean?

Here are some more special terms in the language of hairdressing:

reception The area where clients are received; the process of receiving people.

verbal communication Using words to communicate – talking and writing.

non-verbal communication Using body language to communicate – the way you stand, look and act.

information Knowledge; facts.

consultation The process of interviewing a client.

salon services What the salon offers – cutting, perming, colouring, and the rest.

appointment card A card given to the customer which confirms details of her appointment.

Assignments

1 Describe the duties of a salon receptionist. In particular, make clear in your notes (a) the differences between good and poor communication; (b) situations that should be referred to other members of staff.
   Collect examples of appointment sheets, messages, telephone logs and the like, and add them to your folder.

2 What is your salon's procedure for taking messages?

3 Describe your salon's policy for making appointments.

4 Make a list of the services available at your salon, and their costs.

ACTIVITIES

● Find out which hairdressing services your salon offers. Which ones does the salon specialise in?

● How much do telephone calls cost? Check costs for local and long-distance calls, and calls at different times of the day.

● When you make an appointment, be sure to write down all the details required by both you and the stylist.

Word search

The 10 words listed below are hidden in the diagram.

They have been printed across (backwards or forwards), up or down, or diagonally, but always in a straight line. You can use the letters in the diagram more than once. Can you find them all?

COMMUNICATION
INFORMATION
APPOINTMENT
PRODUCTS
PRICES
CONFIDENTIAL
TELEPHONE
MESSAGES
SMART
ENQUIRIES

Q	M	S	J	W	K	T	M	Y	T	C	N	F	C	X
U	F	E	N	Q	U	I	R	I	E	S	R	O	F	G
A	I	Q	S	E	P	C	E	A	I	X	M	T	R	H
I	N	H	H	I	Q	U	R	C	F	M	X	A	F	K
S	F	N	W	D	Y	Z	Y	O	U	F	U	J	R	T
W	O	F	A	P	P	O	I	N	T	M	E	N	T	T
Y	R	S	V	N	W	G	I	F	A	E	U	L	B	E
S	M	T	U	V	O	C	E	I	O	S	Q	S	U	L
M	A	C	I	E	A	F	R	D	T	S	K	E	Y	E
A	T	U	L	T	E	K	I	E	X	A	J	U	R	P
S	I	D	I	B	U	F	J	N	I	G	T	R	E	H
T	O	O	K	Y	R	D	G	T	D	E	E	A	A	O
I	N	R	A	E	I	A	L	I	E	S	Z	T	E	N
T	Y	P	R	I	C	E	S	A	T	M	B	S	F	E
H	M	I	T	D	I	T	W	L	T	W	W	T	A	A

Multiple-choice questions

1 Which of these should always be carried out before any hairdressing takes place?
a shampooing
b skin testing
c consultation

2 The following is an example of non-verbal communication:
a explanation
b eye contact
c discussion

3 Which service is ideally booked for the early morning or early afternoon?
a CPW
b B/D
c CS/S

Work relationships

To be successful, hairdressers today need a range of abilities and knowledge. They need good all-round technical skills, and a flair for artistic and creative interpretation. They also need to be good communicators. Above all, they must be able to work with others as a team, sharing duties and responsibilities.

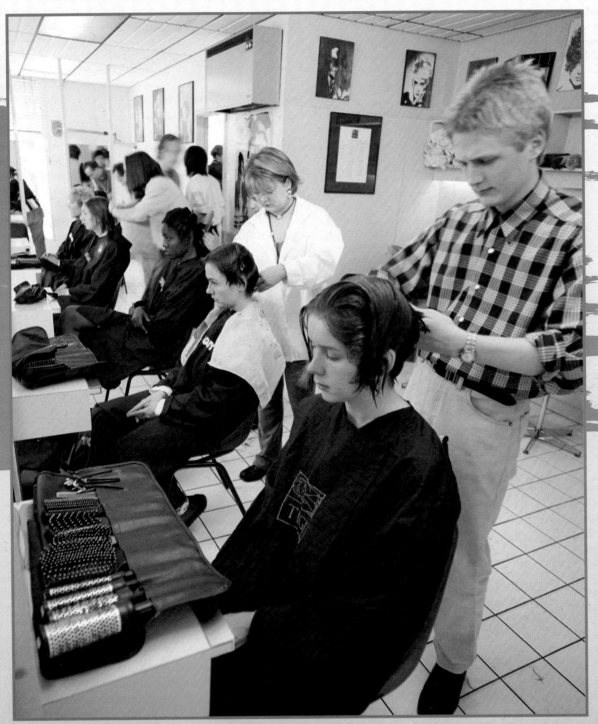

Toni & Guy / Hairdressers Journal

Caring for customers

Caring for customers means doing everything that you can to make the customer happy and comfortable during her visit to the salon.

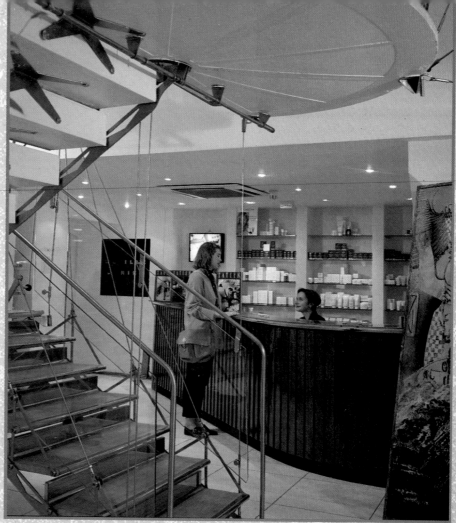

Neville Daniel

What's going on?

Hairdressing is a personal service. A salon's future success is built on developing good communication between all those involved, high levels of technical ability, and high-quality customer service. When a salon achieves this combination, it will earn a good name, and customers will:

● be happy to pay for the services and treatments the salon provides

● keep coming back to the salon

● prefer to buy professional products as advised by the salon

● recommend the salon to their friends and relatives.

All the staff must work together as a team. Everyone has an important role to play, whether as a manager or a shampooist, a stylist or an assistant.

Good customer communication

Good communication is essential if you are to create a good impression and portray the right image. The customer will not just be listening to *what* you are saying but also *how* you say things – your manner, and the tone of your voice. This is especially important in handling enquiries on the telephone.

Think about what *you* would want if *you* were the customer. You would want assistants to be friendly and helpful, and to be able to provide you with accurate information. When you asked for assistance you would expect to be treated courteously and with interest. If the assistant could not help you with your enquiry, you would want to be directed immediately to

someone else who could.

It is not just what is said that communicates information. Your mannerisms and the way you move and hold your body also send out messages. Imagine arriving at the reception of a salon to find the receptionist looking scruffy and bored, seemingly far too busy chatting with someone else to attend to *your* needs. What would you think? First impressions of a salon and its staff are crucial. They create a public image, and this is what the customer will pass on to other people. You need to create a good impression, not just to look after this customer but also to attract the people she knows.

Looking after customers' personal belongings

When a customer arrives at the salon you can assist the receptionist by taking care of her personal belongings. The salon's working area must be kept free of hats, coats, bags and the like: these must be stored safely and securely away from the busy styling and washing areas. Hairdressers use chemicals routinely: the customer's clothes must be protected from accidental spillages of colour, perm solution or bleach. If a client's personal belongings are stolen or accidently damaged, whose fault will it be?

Tips

▮▮▮▮▮▮▮ You will learn more about the job if you:
- watch how others carry out their job
- ask questions and seek advice
- take part in the day-to-day activities.

Simple rules for maintaining good spoken communication

When should you speak to customers?

- When they first enter the salon, during salon services and treatments, and when they need assistance.

What should you say to customers?

- You can ask how you can be of service, you can show interest in their well-being, you can offer refreshments, and you can talk about the products you are using.

How should you speak to customers?

- Always in a courteous, polite manner.

Working as a team

Working together as a team means that everybody contributes, the whole staff sharing the work load. It is important that you listen to your colleagues and follow their instructions: this will save you from wasting time and effort, and will protect you from potential dangers.

Together the team is responsible for maintaining the salon's expected standards of service. Team members can contribute in a variety of ways. Here are some examples.

You can prepare:
- hairdressing tools
- hairdressing equipment
- styling units
- retail displays
- the shampooing area
- client records
- the reception area.

You can assist others by:
- shampooing hair
- conditioning hair
- colour removal
- neutralising hair
- drying hair
- helping at reception
- helping with stock.

You can clear away after:
- perms
- colouring
- cutting services
- salon treatments
- styling services
- clients' departures
- stock deliveries
- product usage.

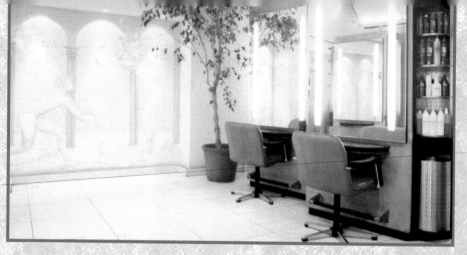

Neville Daniel

Providing support to the team

You can learn more about hairdressing by watching closely how stylists and trainees carry out their day-to-day work. As you 'pass up' rollers or perm curlers you will be able to watch how the stylist's hands and fingers move, manipulating the hair into position. You will be able to give assistance like this in a variety of ways; as you assist you will be able to learn more about styling hair, colouring hair, perming hair, blow-drying hair and cutting hair. Gradually, as you become more familiar with the work, you will learn how to assist without waiting to be asked.

Working in harmony

Working closely as a team will often prevent pressures and stress, but even so there will be times when it will be hard to contain your feelings. Remember, though, that during working hours you are on public display. Whatever your personal feelings towards others, the customers must never sense friction or a bad atmosphere between members of the salon's staff.

You will spend a lot of time in the company of your work associates, and perhaps you will not like everyone all of the time. This should not interfere with the mutual respect to be expected between professional staff at work, which is quite different from what you may be used to in close friendships developed outside work.

Hairdressing preparations

Checklist for preparing customers prior to treatment:

1 Meet and greet each customer in a friendly, courteous way.
2 Check her name and appointment details and confirm that these are correct.
3 Take care of personal items such as hats, coats, jackets or bags.
4 Show the customer to a suitable waiting area.
5 Inform the appropriate stylist of the customer's arrival.
6 Select clean towels and a gown.
7 Find the appropriate service history, or other customer record.

Checklist for preparing the work area:

1 Clean, wipe and tidy the work surfaces, the mirror glass and the foot rest.

2 Dust, tidy and rearrange used hair products.
3 Tidy and put away safely equipment that has been used.
4 Dust down and wipe over the seat, making sure that it is clean and dry.
5 Sweep and clean the floor, ensuring that it is free from cut hair and dirt, and that it is not left wet.

Tips

▭▭▭ Always switch off and unplug electrical equipment when not needed.
▭▭▭ Wipe flexes and leads with a damp cloth and coil them up tidily.
▭▭▭ Wipe exposed metal areas using a general-purpose spray cleaner. Dry them thoroughly, without leaving smears.

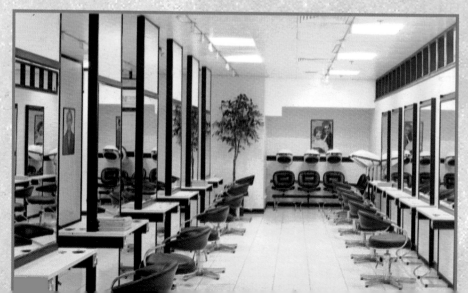

Regis

Improving yourself at work

As you watch your colleagues at work you will notice that they are all doing different things. You can learn from them.

Consider the following activities carried out at reception:
● welcoming customers
● demonstrating and offering goods
● selling products
● accepting payment
● updating customer records
● arranging and displaying products.

Each of these activities involves a variety of tasks. For example, arranging the product displays might include:
● checking the display each morning
● pricing and labelling products
● setting up promotional material
● replacing sold items.

Each of these tasks may be carried out well, adequately, or even badly, depending on the individual's knowledge, skill and attitude.

Knowledge about products could include details of their
● quality
● price
● colour
● size
● availability
● directions for use
● customer benefits.

Skills could include:
● greeting people and making them welcome
● answering questions

● taking money and giving change
● handling other payment types.

Good attitudes at reception towards work could include being
● positive and polite
● courteous and helpful.

What does it mean?

Here are some more special terms in the language of hairdressing.

communication The process of giving and receiving information.
oral communication Using words to communicate – talking and writing.
non-verbal communication Using body language to communicate – the way you stand, look and act.
visual communication Part of non-verbal communication: how you look, and so what the customer sees – and the impressions created by what she sees.
mannerisms Habitual ways of speaking or listening and habitual ways of moving your face or body. Often we are unaware of our own mannerisms.
tone of voice The way in which you speak, which affects the impression you create – loud and harsh tones irritate, quiet and soft tones soothe.

Tips

▦ Make sure that only clean fresh towels and gowns are used.

▦ Clean plastic combs, curlers and perm rods. First make sure that they are free of hair; then scrub with a brush, using detergent and hot water.

▦ Remove hair and dirt from brushes. Wooden brushes can be washed, but should not be left wet. Plastic brushes can be washed in the same way as plastic combs.

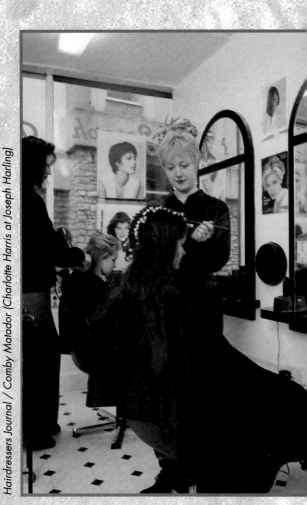

Hairdressers Journal / Comby Matador (Charlotte Harris at Joseph Harling)

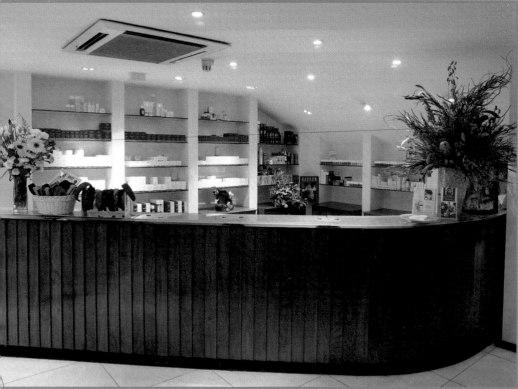

Neville Daniel

Assignments

1 How can you tell whether customers are comfortable and satisfied during their salon visit?

2 What is salon confidentiality? Why is it important to be discreet?

3 Explain in your own words, and with illustrations if you wish, your duties and responsibilities at work. Make special reference to your working relationships with your colleagues.

4 Write down *five* things that you do well, and *five* things that things that you are not so good at. This will help to you identify your strengths and weaknesses. (Keep these in your folder, and review them in a few weeks' time.)

Simple rules for maintaining good visual communication

What do customers want to see?
● Friendly, helpful staff, in a clean and tidy salon: organised, professional people going about their duties.

How should you appear at work?
● Clean, tidy, and smartly dressed; organised and eager to help.

Examples of good and poor service

Good service
● Looking for opportunities to improve the client's comfort and satisfaction during her visit.
● Listening to the customer's requests, comments or concerns.
● Finding out how you can make the customer's visit more comfortable and enjoyable.
● Treating private matters with confidentiality and respect, repeating overheard information only to authorised people.

Poor service
● Not responding to situations where a customer is obviously in need of assistance.
● Ignoring requests from customers.
● Not contributing to the overall salon service requirements.
● Uncaring attitudes towards work and people.

Word search

The 10 words listed below are hidden in the diagram.
They have been printed across (backwards or forwards), up or down,
or diagonally, but always in a straight line. You can use the letters in the
diagram more than once. Can you find them all?

A	J	M	D	N	R	Y	A	H	S	H	W	I	F	T
P	C	I	T	A	X	S	P	R	O	G	R	E	S	S
I	O	H	W	P	H	T	S	B	E	W	Q	J	B	A
H	N	K	I	R	H	O	A	E	P	F	M	O	L	B
M	D	E	T	E	A	M	W	O	R	K	O	B	I	A
E	U	B	F	P	V	P	X	Y	L	V	P	P	C	L
W	C	W	R	A	A	E	C	I	N	I	U	A	S	I
L	T	E	I	R	C	A	M	O	O	H	R	D	H	P
A	X	E	O	E	H	C	D	E	N	I	O	G	M	L
N	W	U	U	P	I	K	U	J	N	Z	T	T	R	S
O	E	Q	D	S	M	P	O	G	E	T	A	R	E	S
S	T	A	N	D	A	R	D	S	F	A	S	F	V	Q
R	T	S	L	W	Q	H	U	N	S	E	E	T	I	Q
E	Y	T	I	L	I	B	I	S	N	O	P	S	E	R
P	E	S	T	W	E	N	E	A	L	E	X	B	W	S

CARING
REVIEW
PROGRESS
TEAMWORK
PREPARE
STANDARDS
PERSONAL
RESPONSIBILITY
ACHIEVEMENT
CONDUCT

Multiple-choice questions

1 Why should we look after customers' belongings?
a because customers are not capable of looking after their own things
b because we are responsible for their safety and security
c so that we can see what they have brought with them

2 What does salon preparation involve?
a waiting to be told to do something
b looking for things that need to be done
c avoiding tasks that need to be done

3 How can your progress be properly reviewed?
a by someone outside the business
b by comparing your efforts against other staff
c by measuring your efforts against previously agreed targets

The salon's resources

The day-to-day movement and management of stock are very important aspects of salon work. Stock control involves a range of activities such as handling, unpacking, counting, storing, stacking and checking, and product display. Many of these duties will be new to you: the following pages explain why these duties are so important and how to carry them out safely.

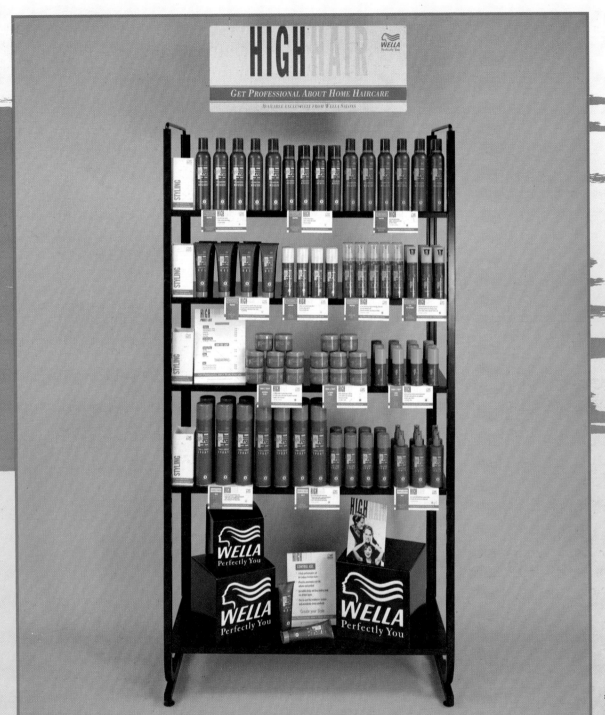

Checking stock

Every salon needs a certain amount of stock so that it can function normally. Imagine that a customer is arriving today at 10.00 for a perm. To carry out the perm someone will have to make sure beforehand that:
● enough curlers of the correct sizes are available
● combs, clips and scissors are to hand
● protective items such as towels, gowns, capes, cottonwool and gloves are available
● stocks of shampoo, conditioner and perming chemicals are sufficient.

The specific amounts of these items normally held will vary from salon to salon. Each salon will decide the *minimum holding level* that will allow the salon to provide the various services and treatments it offers. If stocks fall below these levels, sales may be lost.

Salon staff make checks on the stock regularly, to monitor both the quantity and the quality of the products.

Checking the quantity

The amount of stock, whether in storage or on display, must be accurately counted. This can be quite difficult as not all stock items

What's going on?

You need to know what the salon's resources are, and how to make the best use of them. The term *resources* refers to the products, the tools and items of equipment, and the utilities such as power and water. These all need to be used, handled and displayed properly.
● Tools and equipment must be handled safely and correctly so that you don't put at risk the health and safety of yourself or anyone else.
● Products must be displayed to their best advantage so that they can easily be seen, generating sales for the salon.
● Equipment, power and water must be used in ways which minimise wastage and maximise cost-effectiveness.

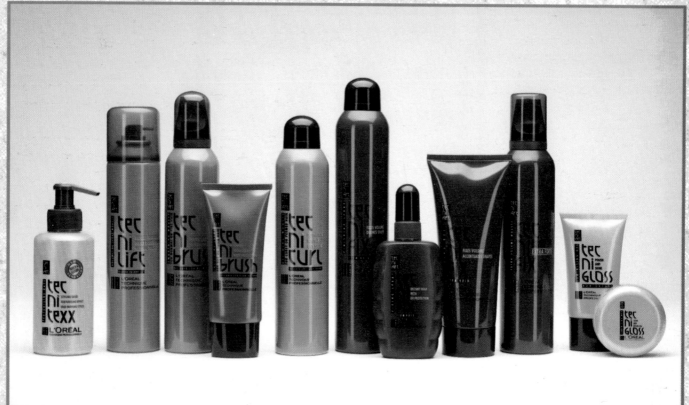

L'Oréal

are sold as single units. You will need to find out from your supervisor:

● How are items counted? (Are they single units, sets, multiples or packs?)
● Who is the manufacturer (e.g. Wella, Goldwell or L'Oréal)?
● What is the product category? (Is it a perm or a shampoo; combs, scissors or curlers?)
● What type of product is it? (Is the product for a particular hair type, or does it have special uses?)

Checking the quality

During normal stock control procedures, the product quality – its condition – will be checked at the same time as product counting. Whenever new stock is delivered to the salon, the same rules apply.

All goods are required by law to be sold to an expected standard ('saleable condition'). Any goods falling short of this, either through deterioration or through damage, must be identified and reported immediately. Product damage or deterioration could occur through:

● a manufacturing process (during the making)
● transportation (during the process of delivery)
● incorrect or poor handling
● unsuitable storage conditions.

If stock is damaged or in poor condition when it is delivered, it must not be accepted. You should report problems to your manager at once.

Stock records

Each salon adopts its own system for documenting the movements of stock. These records must be accurate and up to date. The diagram shows the various stages of stock management.

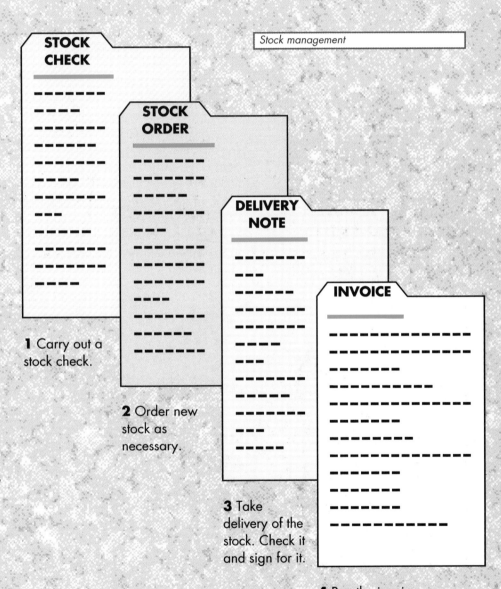

Stock management

STOCK CHECK

STOCK ORDER

DELIVERY NOTE

INVOICE

1 Carry out a stock check.

2 Order new stock as necessary.

3 Take delivery of the stock. Check it and sign for it.

4 Pay the invoice.

Stock arriving at the salon

receipt. Before the goods can be signed for, however, the contents of the boxes and packages must be checked against the delivery note to make sure that nothing is missing, that nothing is damaged, and that nothing has deteriorated.

Stock ordered from a manufacturer is delivered direct to the salon by road carrier, whereas supplies ordered from a local wholesaler will usually be collected in person. In either event, when the stock arrives at reception it will need to be moved into storage as soon as possible.

Handling stock the right way

Handling stock involves physical work in lifting and carrying. This must be done safely, to minimise the risk of injury. (See page 59.)

First look at the outside of the packaging. What are the contents? Are there are any special handling conditions? Below are some examples of such handling instructions.

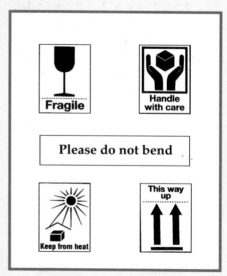

Unpacking stock the right way

Supplies arrive in a variety of boxes and other types of packaging. Boxes may have special bindings, seals and staples, or strong adhesive tapes. Packages may be coated in shrink-fit plastic, vacuum-sealed, tied, or bubble-wrapped. Watch others to see how they unpack goods without damaging them, and also without causing injury to themselves.

The delivery note

An itemised delivery note will accompany the goods received. This will show:

● the date of dispatch
● the sender's name and address
● details of the contents
● any goods marked 'out of stock' or 'to follow'
● the delivery name and address.

The person who delivers the goods will require a signature as proof of

The stock replacement cycle

This diagram shows the continuing stock-control process.

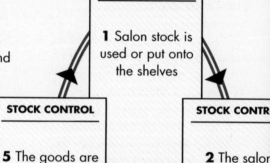

STOCK CONTROL

1 Salon stock is used or put onto the shelves

STOCK CONTROL

5 The goods are received and signed for

STOCK CONTR

2 The salon stock is check

STOCK CONTROL

4 Replacement stock is ordered

STOCK CONTROL

3 Some items are below the minimum holding level

Storing stock properly

Handling

Handling and lifting goods can be dangerous. You must not move items unless you have had appropriate training. If a box or package seems heavy or awkward, do not attempt to lift it. Instead, tell your supervisor immediately.

The following guidance about manual handling is adapted from information supplied by the Health and Safety Executive:

1 *Stop and think about what you are going to do* Plan the lift. Where are you going to put the load? Use appropriate aids if possible. Do you need help with the load? Remove any obstructions, such as discarded wrapping materials. Plan to lift with the heaviest side of the load close to your body. If you cannot get close enough to it, try sliding it towards you before you attempt to lift it. For a long lift – such as from the floor to shoulder height – consider resting the load half-way, perhaps on a table, so that you can change your grip.

2 *Place your feet carefully* Stand with your feet apart, as this gives a balanced and stable base while lifting. (A tight skirt or unsuitable footwear will make this difficult.) Put the leading leg as far forward as is comfortable.

3 *Adopt a good posture* Bend your knees so that when you grasp the load, your hands are as near as possible level with your waist. (However, do not kneel or overflex your knees.) Keep your back straight. Lean forward over the load, if necessary, to get a good grip. Keep your shoulders level, and facing in the same direction as your hips.

4 *Get a firm grip* Try to keep your arms within the boundary formed by your legs. The best position for holding the load, and how you hold it, depend on circumstances. Be sure that you have a secure grip.

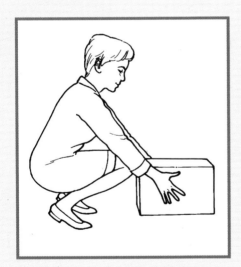

5 *Don't jerk* Carry out the lifting movement smoothly. Keep control of the load.

6 *Move your feet* When turning to the side, move your feet – don't twist your trunk.

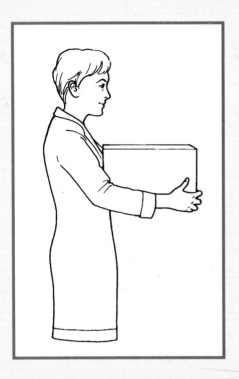

7 *Keep close to the load* Keep the load close to the body for as long as you can.

8 *Put the load down, then adjust its position* If you need to put the load in a precise position, put it down first and then *slide* it into position.

Storage

The majority of salon stock should be kept in a secure, locked location. The area should contain shelves that can be adjusted, allowing packages and boxes of varying sizes to be stored properly. Products should be stored upright to avoid leakage or spillage, and should not be stacked on top of each other. The size of the storage space will depend on the salon's needs – it might be a whole room or just a cupboard.

Displaying stock correctly

Hairdressing salons take special care when displaying their products. The aim is to encourage customers to talk about the products and then buy them, generating income for the salon. Therefore:

● products must be clearly visible
● product information must be readily to hand
● displays must be clean, attractive and inviting
● product condition and quality must be carefully monitored.

Product promotion is the most important aspect of salon retailing. While customers are having their hair done, the stylist can talk about the products she is using. Also, customers need advice on how to look after their hairstyles: they will want to know how they can achieve similar effects when they look after their own hair at home.

The salon can back up the promotion with attractive *retail displays*; in reception, in front windows, and around the salon. These contribute to the professional image that the salon portrays to the public. Products left on shelves, however, will over time gather dust. Both the products and the shelves will therefore need regular cleaning. You can encourage customers to pick up and handle the products, to read the product information and to smell the fragrance. They will not want to touch dirty products on murky shelves!

In addition to cleaning, other duties will include monitoring the amount and condition of the stock. Unless products are available you cannot sell them, so someone needs to check daily to find out whether any items need replacing.

Some products have a limited *shelf life*; as with food in supermarkets, items may have a 'sell by' or 'use by' date. When stock needs replacing, take particular care to bring older products to the front of the shelves, and put newer, more recent stock arrivals at the back. This process is commonly known as *stock rotation*.

L'Oréal

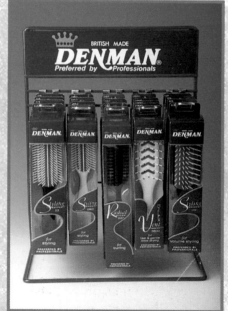

Denman

Security of stock

Stock is a valuable asset for the salon. A salon which has an accurate stock-control system will be able to spot incorrect records or shortages promptly.

Theft during business hours by visitors to the salon can be minimised if staff are trained to check the identity of callers. If you approach someone who is acting suspiciously, and they do not give you a satisfactory explanation of their visit, alert a senior member of staff immediately. Do not put yourself at any risk. If the individual runs away, the incident will need to be reported to the police. You may then be called to give an account of what took place, and you will be asked for:

● the date and time of the incident
● an account of what actually took place
● a description of the intruder.

Unfortunately, salon visitors are not the only people who may steal salon property. Theft by staff – often referred to as 'shrinkage' – may also occur. Whoever takes them, the unauthorised taking of money, goods or equipment is always classed as theft. Thefts by staff members are considered acts of gross misconduct, and can lead to disciplinary procedures or to instant dismissal.

Minimising waste

Salons need to be cost-effective if they are to remain profitable. Wasting resources is simply throwing money away.

Colour and curl chemicals

Most of the chemical products used in the salon today come prepacked, ready to use. Nevertheless, the amounts used for individual clients may vary, so it is important to be careful and accurate in measuring

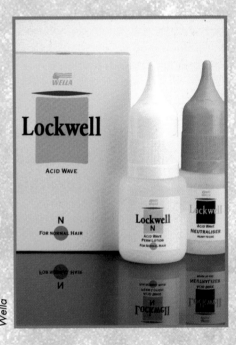

Wella

them. These chemicals include perm solutions, neutraliser, hair-colouring products and bleaches.

Cleansing and conditioning

Shampoos and conditioners are often used directly from bulk sizes, so it is quite easy to overestimate the amounts needed. If you do, you will be rinsing the products and profits down the basin!

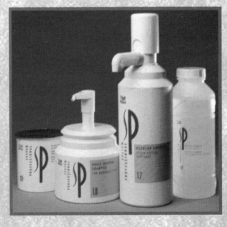

Wella

Styling and fixing products

The styling and fixing products used in the modern salon include a wide range of mousses, gels, waxes and hair-fixing sprays. These items are used directly from their containers. Take care not to use more than is needed on the customer's hair. Overloading the hair with these products is a waste of both time and money: it also makes styling difficult or impossible.

Tools and equipment

Be sure to use the salon's equipment as intended by the manufacturer. Misuse of equipment or incorrect handling are the main reasons for damage. Repairs can be very expensive. Consider, for example, modern high-quality scissors which can cost anything between £10 and £400. These are precision-made tools. If dropped on the floor or used for cutting anything other than hair, the machined edges could be damaged beyond satisfactory repair.

Particular care and attention is required also in cleaning and maintaining salon equipment.

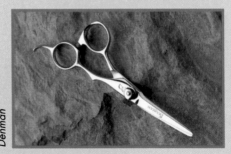

Denman

Water and power

Water is a valuable resource. Turn the taps off between shampooing and conditioning, and avoid excessive rinsing during neutralising – unnecessary use of water is a waste of money. To save electricity, turn off heaters in the staff room when not required, and lights in areas of the salon that are not being used. Run hood dryers only as long as necessary.

Telecommunications

Unless a separate telephone is provided in your salon, do not use the salon phone for personal calls. The business line is the salon's lifeline to customers: it must be left clear for incoming calls. Remember also that unauthorised calls made at the salon's expense could be classed as theft.

Assignments

1 Describe, with illustrations, the system your salon uses in maintaining stock control. Make special reference to counting the levels of stock, replacing stock, stock rotation, and the relevant health and safety issues. (Add your notes to your folder.)

2 Give reasons for minimising wastage, referring to products, power, water, the telephone, and time.

3 What are the possible consequences of using the above resources incorrectly?

What does it mean?

Here are some more special terms in the language of hairdressing.

resources Tools (e.g. scissors), products (e.g. shampoo), and services (e.g. water).

stock Materials or goods for sale or for use in the salon.

products or goods Items of stock.

stock records Detailed lists of goods for sale or for use in the salon.

stock check The process of checking the quantity and quality of goods.

deterioration Damage to, or spoilage of, stored goods.

delivery note A written record of the details of goods delivered.

Word search

The 10 words listed below are hidden in the diagram.
They have been printed across (backwards or forwards), up or down,
or diagonally, but always in a straight line. You can use the letters in the
diagram more than once. Can you find them all?

RESOURCES
POWER
STOCK
EQUIPMENT
QUANTITY
RECORDS
REPLACEMENT
DELIVERY
ORDER
STORAGE

I	F	R	H	S	O	I	P	J	G	D	B	O	O	V
E	T	N	E	M	P	I	U	Q	E	F	R	O	A	E
B	R	E	D	R	O	S	B	U	S	H	A	R	Y	G
I	T	A	G	T	I	B	C	D	V	A	R	H	S	I
N	F	I	W	T	S	T	R	A	N	F	B	D	W	K
W	O	P	O	B	L	O	B	P	L	T	A	S	T	P
F	N	T	R	B	C	N	E	S	P	R	D	Z	S	Y
L	U	W	R	E	P	L	A	C	E	M	E	N	T	S
U	E	N	R	O	W	A	I	F	N	O	L	C	O	O
G	G	S	S	M	T	O	A	T	O	Y	I	E	C	C
L	A	D	H	K	A	L	P	T	P	L	V	V	K	H
B	R	E	S	O	U	R	C	E	S	P	E	I	I	P
M	O	J	C	M	O	I	D	P	K	O	R	L	O	L
X	T	D	R	Q	U	A	N	T	I	T	Y	T	H	U
O	S	W	O	T	S	T	W	O	B	Z	W	F	D	X

Multiple-choice questions

1 Why do salons buy stock?
a to fill up empty shelves
b for the staff's own needs
c to use on, or to resell to, customers

2 Why is it important to minimise wastage?
a to be more cost-effective
b to please managers
c to meet health and safety regulations

3 What form arrives with stock?
a a delivery note
b an invoice
c a stock order

Personal health and work safety

Hairdressers have a responsibility to the members of the public they serve: we must take care of ourselves, and we must consider the health and safety of others.

We are legally bound to do this.

This chapter looks closely at the health and safety issues that affect you at work. In particular, we shall look at personal health, hygiene, and working safely.

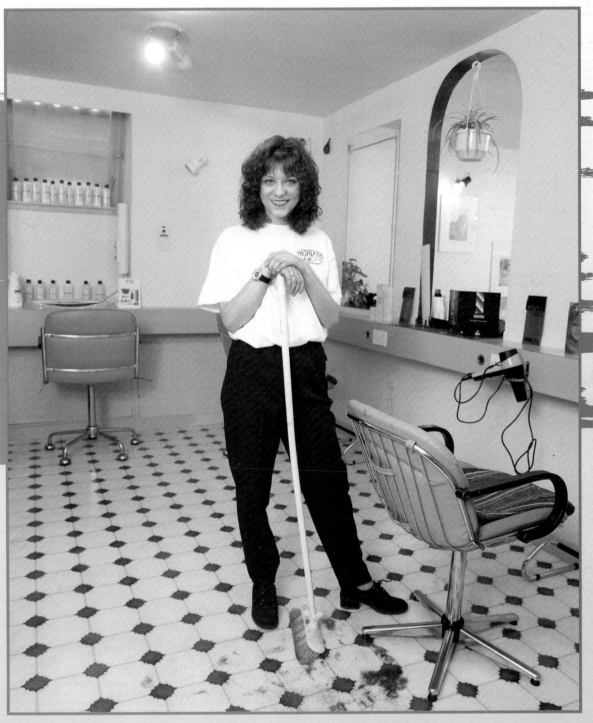

Hairdressers Journal / Comby Matador (Laura Davies at Highland Hair Studio)

Health and hygiene

Hand and nail care

You will be using your hands to style, massage and manipulate your customer's hair, so your hands and nails must be scrupulously clean. If your hands are dirty or your nails unclean, they may harbour bacteria. These can spread to other people (*cross-infection*). Your hands will need washing many times throughout the day.

● Always wash them *after* handling waste items, after general salon maintenance, and after using the lavatory.
● Always wash them *before* handling food or touching clients' hair.

During washing and shampooing your hands come into contact with detergents. Repeated contact with chemical detergents will remove the skin's natural moisture and suppleness. This will lead to dryness and chapped or cracked skin, which allows germs to enter and may cause infection. Repeated exposure to detergents and other cleansing agents may also lead to dermatitis, a skin condition which 'reddens' the skin, making it sore or painful; cracks may result, often accompanied by itching.

To prevent dermatitis, you must ensure that your hands are dried properly each time after washing. You should then apply a suitable *barrier cream*: this covers the skin with an invisible protective layer, greatly reducing the penetration of hairdressing preparations. In

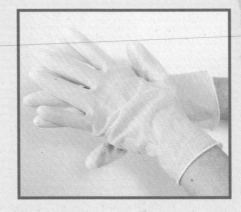

situations where your hands are exposed to stronger chemicals, you should always wear rubber gloves.

Your nails should be well manicured and not too long. Long nails will not only trap dirt underneath them, but may also cause discomfort to clients. It is difficult to shampoo correctly if your nails are long: the nails will prevent you from massaging the scalp correctly without scratching it, and may also tangle in longer hair.

A clean body

Regular washing is essential – take a bath or shower every day. This will remove sweat, dead skin cells and surface bacteria. By ensuring that your body is clean you can be confident of preventing body odour. *Anti-perspirants* reduce underarm sweating. These products contain *astringents*, chemicals that narrow the pores (through which come perspiration which cools down the skin). *Deodorants* simply mask any odour by killing the surface bacteria: they do not reduce the amount of perspiration.

Fresh breath

Bad breath is offensive to clients: it is important to prevent this. When we have bad breath, we may not be aware of it ourselves. It usually results from tiny particles of food left to decay in the spaces between our teeth: that is why it is important to brush your teeth after meals. However, it can also result from digestive troubles, stomach upsets, smoking, and strong foods such as onions, garlic, curries and some cheeses. If you are prone to having bad breath (some people are), use an antiseptic mouthwash after cleaning your teeth.

Good posture

Bad posture will lead to fatigue or possibly to a longer-term injury. It is essential to adopt the correct posture. An incorrect standing position will not only put undue strain on your muscles and ligaments; it will also give customers the impression that you are uncaring and unprofessional in your work.

Personal appearance

As well as being clean, you need to think about your appearance. Let the time and effort you put into getting ready for work reflect your pride in your job. A customer can easily tell the difference between a staff member who allowed plenty of time to get ready and one who has arrived just in the nick of time after getting up late or oversleeping.

You can choose the way you look, provided that you take into account the standards of dress and appearance expected by your salon.

Clothes

Clothes or overalls should be clean and well ironed. Wear clothes made from fabrics suited to your work and to the time of year. Avoid clothes that are restrictive or tight: you will want air to be able to circulate around your body to keep you cool and fresh. It's not just external clothes that matter: clean underwear is essential too.

Footwear

Wear shoes with low heels. They should be smart and comfortable, and made of materials suitable for wearing over long periods of time. Hairdressing involves a lot of standing – your feet can get tired, hot, sweaty and even sore. It is worth wearing shoes that allow your feet to 'breathe', so that they remain cool and comfortable throughout the working day.

Hair and hairstyle

Your hair naturally reflects the image and the standards of the salon in which you work. Your hair should be clean, healthy and manageable. Don't let long hair fall over your face where it would obstruct good communication with customers.

Working safely

Hazards and potential hazards

What is a hazard? One dictionary definition is 'exposure or vulnerability to injury or loss'. It is the duty of your manager to ensure that your salon is free from hazard.

There is a difference between a hazard and a *potential* hazard. Imagine that you are asked by your employer to clean and prepare an open razor ready for use. Though you have had no previous or appropriate training, you do what

Your jewellery

Only the minimum of jewellery should be worn in the salon. Rings, bracelets and dangling necklaces will get in the way of normal day-to-day duties and will make customers feel uncomfortable. In many hairdressing operations such as shampooing and conditioning, jewellery can easily catch and pull at the customer's hair, as well as providing unhygienic crevices where dirt and germs can lurk.

has been asked and in the process you cut yourself. Your employer is then at fault because she exposed you to a *hazard*.

If before carrying out the task you had received the correct training for cleaning and preparing sharp instruments, you would be exposed to a *potential* hazard – but your training would prevent you from sustaining any injury.

Infections and disease

We all carry large numbers of *micro-organisms* inside us, on our skin and in our hair. These organisms, which include bacteria, fungi and viruses, are too small to be seen with the naked eye. Many micro-organisms are quite harmless, others can cause disease. Those that are harmful to people are called *pathogens*. Flu, for example, is caused by a virus; thrush by a fungus; and bronchitis often by bacteria. Conditions like these which can be transmitted from one person to another are said to be *infectious*.

Our bodies are naturally resistant to infection; they fight most pathogens using an in-built immunity system. So you may carry pathogenic organisms without contracting the associated disease. When you do have a disease, there are visible signs that something is wrong: these are called *symptoms*. Different symptoms help us to recognise different diseases.

Infectious diseases are normally treated by a doctor, whereas non-infectious conditions can often be treated in the salon or with products available from a pharmacist.

Preventing infection

The tools and implements we use in salons must be *hygienic*. As well as the routine cleaning of the salon and its equipment (page 50), smaller pieces of salon equipment may need specialised cleaning processes.

Some salons use sterilising

devices to ensure that their work implements are completely safe from infection. *Sterilisation* means that all living organisms are killed.

Handling chemicals

The services you provide to customers involve the use of many products, which vary in their effects on the customer's hair. Some cleanse the hair and scalp; others condition and moisturise. Some products modify the natural structure of hair or assist in reshaping it; others alter the natural pigments of hair.

All of these products contain chemicals. Many of these chemicals are either acidic or alkaline: depending on their strength, they may be corrosive or caustic, and liable to damage skin.

Government regulations concerning the Control of Substances Hazardous to Health (COSHH) specify details of the safe handling of hazardous chemicals. This information should be posted up in your salon, and particular equipment to be worn with particular chemicals should be available. COSHH rules *must* be followed, to ensure both your safety and the safety of others.

Hazardous chemicals are usually identified on packaging by standard warning symbols, or icons.

HSE
Health & Safety
Executive

COSHH
a brief guide
for employers

The requirements of the Control of Substances Hazardous to Health (COSHH) Regulations 1988

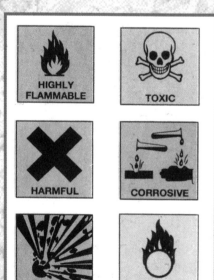

HIGHLY FLAMMABLE · TOXIC · HARMFUL · CORROSIVE · EXPLOSIVE · OXIDIZING

Tip

If you have to clear up spilt chemicals or damaged equipment, take care. What is the substance or item that has been dropped? Is it something that needs special care in handling? Should you be wearing gloves?

Electricity and water

It is not just chemicals that need to be handled safely: care should be taken with other salon resources too, especially electricity and hot water.

Your manager will make sure that all electrical equipment is regularly checked by a qualified person, but even so equipment faults may occur during normal operation. A common problem is that with constant use the leads on items such as hairdryers, clippers and tongs may work loose or become damaged. If you see that this has happened, do not attempt to touch or disconnect the appliance, but tell your supervisor immediately and leave it to her to take the appropriate action.

Hot water is used in all operations carried out at the basin. To avoid any discomfort to customers – or worse, scalding of the skin – always test the temperature of the water on the back of your hand before rinsing the customer's hair. When using shower mixers, always 'build up' the water temperature by slowly decreasing the cold supply at the tap. Never use the shower head without first testing the water temperature.

Obstructions

Obstructions are potential hazards too. It is particularly dangerous to obstruct areas used as thoroughfares – doorways, corridors, stairs and fire exits must always be kept clear. In an emergency, people might have to leave the salon in a hurry, perhaps even in the dark. At such a time an obstruction could be disastrous, causing someone to fall or be injured.

Safe disposal of waste

Everyday items of salon waste should be placed in an enclosed waste bin fitted with a suitably resistant polyethylene bin liner. When the bin is full, seal the liner using a wire tie and place the bag ready for refuse collection. If for any reason the bin liner punctures, put the damaged liner and waste inside a second bin liner. Wash out the bin itself with hot water and detergent.

Disposable items with sharp edges, such as used razor blades, should be placed in a safe screw-topped container. When the container is full it can be disposed of safely. This type of salon waste, known as 'sharps', should be kept separate from general salon waste – special disposal may be required by your local authority. (Contact your local council offices for more information.)

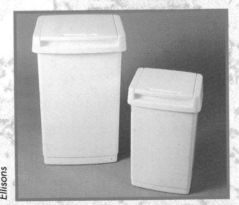

Ellisons

Tip

▮▮▮▮ Always be on the lookout for any obstruction. If you see something that could present a risk, move it away as soon as you can.

Assignments

First aid

When accidents occur in the salon, the designated first-aiders will normally administer the first aid. In situations involving minor accidents, you can assist by treating the patient yourself. You will find a first-aid guidance card in the box containing the first-aid kit.

1 Find out where your salon's first-aid equipment is kept.
2 Make a list of the first-aid items recommended for a standard first-aid box. (Keep this list in your folder.)

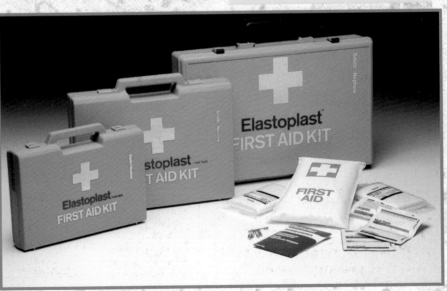

Smith & Nephew, Hull

Assignments

Fire and emergency evacuation

It is essential that you know the fire procedures.

1 Find out your salon's procedures for:
a fire prevention
b raising the alarm
c evacuation during a fire
d assembly points following evacuation.

2 Various fire extinguishers are available, containing different types of fire-fighting materials.
a How many types are there?
b What are their different uses?

What does it mean?

Here are some more special terms in the language of hairdressing.

health hazard A danger to the health or welfare of customers or staff.
potential hazard A possible danger.
germs Small organisms that may cause disease.
pathogenic Able to cause disease.
non-pathogenic Not able to cause disease.
BO Body odour.
posture The way you hold your body.
HSE The Health and Safety Executive.
COSHH The Control of Substances Hazardous to Health regulations.

Assignments

Personal health

1 What are the expected standards at your salon regarding appearance and clothes?
2 How can bad posture affect personal health?
3 What kinds of personal protective equipment might you wear at work? When should you wear them?
4 Explain how infection can spread at work. How can you prevent it from spreading?

5 Explain in your own words why it is important to work safely. Describe some of the possible hazards within a hair salon.
6 Why is it important to carry out regular safety checks at work? What sorts of things should be checked?
7 What are the correct, safe ways of disposing of salon waste?

(Add all of these notes to your folder.)

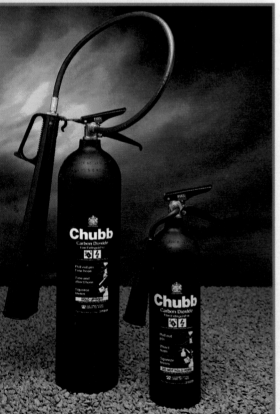

Fire Protection Services

Word search

The 10 words listed below are hidden in the diagram.
They have been printed across (backwards or forwards), up or down,
or diagonally, but always in a straight line. You can use the letters in the
diagram more than once. Can you find them all?

DERMATITIS
HYGIENE
EMERGENCY
APPEARANCE
HAZARD
INFECTION
FIRST AID
STERILISATION
CHEMICALS
WASTE

V	F	C	V	H	E	Z	M	U	J	M	W	L	N	N
S	I	T	I	T	A	M	R	E	D	T	L	E	A	O
P	R	D	U	A	R	Y	A	A	R	K	J	P	R	A
O	S	A	O	O	E	G	N	I	A	I	P	B	P	J
M	T	B	R	E	D	P	E	D	Z	E	N	N	M	T
W	A	S	T	E	E	N	R	I	A	S	N	A	N	A
T	I	T	U	I	E	B	O	R	H	T	U	S	O	W
S	D	T	H	I	P	H	A	A	E	L	R	I	I	H
O	A	Q	G	C	M	N	E	Y	D	Y	R	A	T	L
L	H	Y	D	Y	C	N	E	G	R	E	M	E	C	T
T	H	B	L	E	X	I	H	O	C	H	H	A	E	S
B	I	F	T	K	N	A	P	W	O	L	M	T	F	H
K	S	T	E	R	I	L	I	S	A	T	I	O	N	O
U	A	J	O	O	W	V	P	H	L	L	K	P	I	H
S	L	A	C	I	M	E	H	C	C	J	D	I	E	W

Multiple-choice questions

1 Why should you bother about your
personal appearance at work?
a to compete against your colleagues
b to show that you take pride in your job
c to impress friends who may call in

2 Who is responsible for your safety at
work?
a your parents
b your friends
c you

3 Who should treat infectious diseases?
a the salon manager
b the doctor
c you

Career opportunities in hairdressing

Hairdressing is an exciting industry, offering a career full of opportunities. Have you ever thought about working in the television and film industry, of working on a cruise liner, of becoming a lecturer or of owning your own business?

This chapter gives you an insight into the industry, and will help you find out more about the qualifications, the personal requirements, and the different areas of work available in hairdressing.

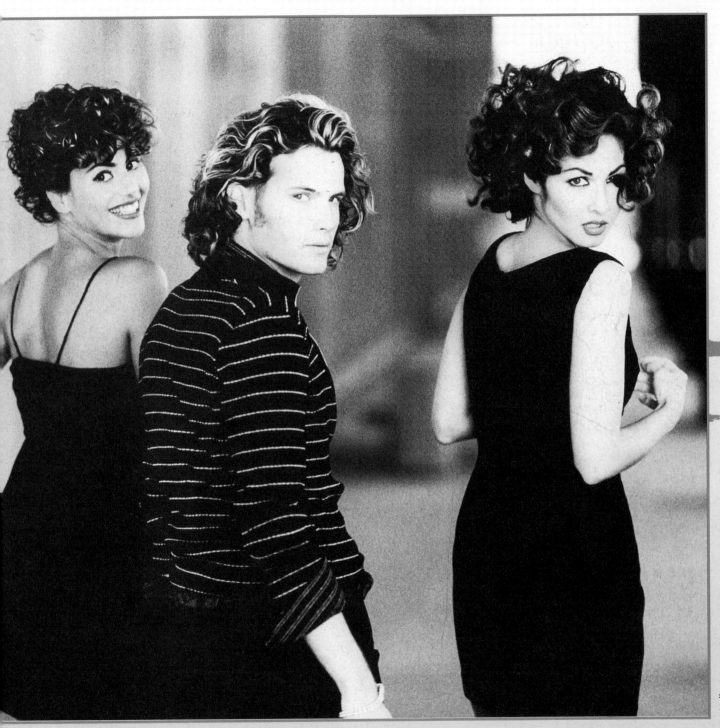

Wella

What is a career?

A career is the course and the purpose of a lifetime's work; it is what you work at from day to day. Nevertheless, your career may change direction, and in time you may work in areas you had never thought about.

In the final year at school there is usually a lot of discussion about what career you might follow. Among your friends no doubt some will know exactly what they want to do, while others may be unsure.

Fortunately such differences between people are well recognised – leaving school is a beginning, not an end. Most training programmes include topics that have general application in a range of jobs, as well as topics specific to a chosen area of work.

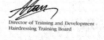

City & Guilds
National
Vocational
Qualification

HAIRDRESSING LEVEL 1

This Certificate
is awarded to   ELMORE QUACKENBUSH

The holder has one or more formal Certificates of Unit Credit
by which this award was earned

Awarded   MARCH 1996   9507/141427/301021/ZZZ9999/M/01/01/01

Director-General
The City and Guilds of London Institute

Director of Training and Development
Hairdressing Training Board

The City and Guilds of London Institute *Incorporated* by Royal Charter *Founded* 1878

Qualifications

Why do you need a qualification?

A qualification demonstrates to other people that you have been trained to do particular work, both safely and well. It is the way that others – your future customers – can be sure that you can be relied upon. To this end, training standards are agreed between the organisations in the hairdressing industry concerned with the preparation of young entrants – trainees, students and apprentices. A variety of people are needed for a wide range of jobs: the training standards ensure that each person can do her job professionally.

The joint awarding body consisting of the Hairdressing Training Board (HTB) and the City &

Guilds of London Institute (CGLI), supported by the Hairdressing Council and other leading hairdressing organisations. This body ensures that the skills of entrants meet the needs of the hairdressing industry. When you meet the introductory standards you can be awarded the National Vocational Qualification (NVQ) or the Scottish Vocational Qualification (SVQ) at Level 1. As you progress, you can attempt Levels 2, 3 and 4.

- **NVQ Level 1** is an introductory level: it allows you to gain some insight into hairdressing as you assist in salons.

- **NVQ Level 2** is the foundational level: it qualifies you to work in salons.

- **NVQ Level 3** is a professional level: all aspects of hairdressing are included and you attain more advanced levels of work.

- **NVQ Level 4** is a management qualification: it allows you to administer salons and manage staff.

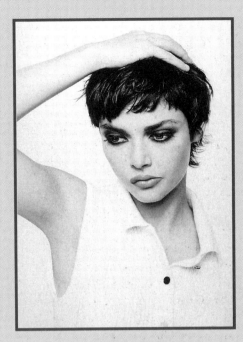

Toni & Guy

Training

Where is hairdressing training carried

Hairdressing salons, private schools, training centres and further education colleges may provide training to meet the needs of the hairdressing industry. Most work to the standards of the HTB and CGLI, and many salons are recognised training centres.

A variety of courses have been designed to meet the needs of all trainees. Apart from the study of the theory and practice of ladies' and men's hairdressing, art, biology and chemistry may also be studied. Related studies in the future may include wigmaking and dressing, manicure, make-up, various aspects of beauty and cosmetics, and training and management skills: these will be part of studies beyond Level 1.

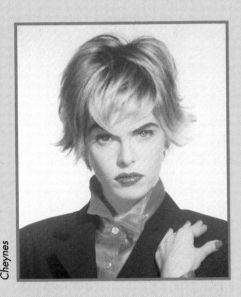

Cheynes

What personal attributes do you need to become a hairdresser?

In hairdressing there are artistic and scientific pathways to be followed – some people are successful in both.

Entrants to hairdressing need the following basic qualities:

- a pleasing personality
- an acceptable appearance
- fitness and good health
- enthusiasm
- patience
- artistic flair
- reliability and punctuality
- the ability to communicate
- efficiency and motivation.

What academic qualifications do you need?

Beginners should ideally have passed exams in English language, mathematics, art and science, but these are not essential.

Areas of work

Where can you work as a hairdresser?

There is a wide variety of jobs to be done in hairdressing, carried out in different places and in different situations. Each job has its own special needs.

The following list includes most hairdressing jobs.

Towns and cities
These have large and small salons, offering a range of services to meet the needs of many regular and passing customers.

Country districts
These have fewer potential customers and are more reliant on a regular clientele.

Seaside and holiday areas
Because of seasonal variations in the numbers of customers, these require special organisation.

Shopping precincts
These are usually sited in busy areas, and again need to cater for fluctuating customer numbers.

Airports and travel terminals
Many of these offer salon services to busy travellers.

Department stores
These meet the needs of customers most of whom have been attracted into the store by other services.

Leisure centres, gymnasiums and health clubs
Many of these now offer salon services.

Hotels
These offer a variety of services to meet the needs of their customers.

Hospitals
These cater for patients' needs: many patients will be bedridden or restricted in their movement.

Professional freelance hairdressing
These hairdressers offer qualified hairdressing in customers' own homes.

Nursing homes
These require special care for customers who may be restricted, disabled or aged.

Hospices
Like nursing homes, these offer hair and beauty services to people with particular needs.

Holiday camps
These deal with changing numbers of customers, according to the season.

Armed forces camps
These usually have their own salon facilities.

Beauty salons
Many offer hairdressing services also, to meet their customers' needs.

Hair and scalp clinics
These are special clinics offering hair care and trichological treatments.

Prisons
These cater for prisoners' needs.

Cruise liners
These meet the needs of the ship's passengers.

Television studios
These deal with the varied needs of presenters, interviewers and actors.

Theatrical studios
Usually these offer wigmaking as well as hairdressing services.

Film and photographic studios
In these fashion, high fashion and creative hairdressing are required.

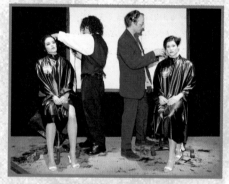

Mahogany

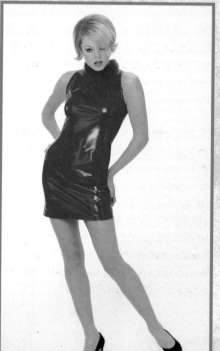

TRESemmé

What careers are available within the world of hairdressing?

Hairdressing salons are of varying types and sizes. They may be individual salons, catering for special needs or offering particular skills and services, or they may be part of a large group, offering a wide range of hairdressing services. Some may offer fashion cutting, specialised colouring or creative hair styling for which special training and experience are required. The following list shows some of the many careers open to you.

● *Hairdressers* are trained and qualified in general hairdressing techniques, and have both technical ability and artistic flair.
● *Hair stylists* are usually hairdressers who specialise in fashioning hair dressings, shapes and styles. The creative and artistic hair stylist – someone who is able to be original – is always in demand.
● *Receptionists* deal with people, making appointments, answering enquiries and handling payments. Good communication, organisational and presentational skills are required.
● *Technicians* specialise in one or more hairdressing techniques (e.g. perming or colouring), but are not necessarily adept in all hairdressing skills.
● *Colourists* specialise in colour choice and in the application of all colouring techniques, working closely with hairdressers and stylists.
● *Permers* specialise in the choice and application of all perming techniques, working closely with hairdressers and stylists.
● *Blow dryers* and *blow setters* offer the special skills and techniques of hair drying and setting.
● *Shampooists* are employed especially to shampoo customers in the salon.
● *Cutters* offer special cutting skills and techniques in addition to general hairdressing skills.
● *Owner stylists* both manage their salons and work in them, styling and so on.
● *Owner managers* offer management skills, but do not themselves carry out hairdressing.
● *Managers and co-assistant managers* may be employed (mainly by larger salons) to co-ordinate the artistic, technical and management skills of the staff.

Some other routes to success

Not all career routes confine you to the salon: some allow you to travel and spend considerable time away. The following are some of the possibilities.

● *Hairdressing consultants* advise and guide other salon organisations.
● *Demonstrators* offer product knowledge and technical and artistic hairdressing. They have special presentational skills and are employed particularly by leading colour and wholesale suppliers.
● *Competition workers* deal with a range of artistic hairdressing, events, displays and shows.
● *Hairdressing representatives* and *technical advisers* offer product knowledge and scientific advice to salon staff.
● *Teachers* and *lecturers* train others in colleges and schools.
● *Trainers* work in salons, colleges and schools.
● *Salon owners* run their own salon, or a chain or group of salons.
● *Trichologists* specialise in hair and skin conditions. They may operate a hair or beauty salon themselves or work as consultants in private practice, or both.

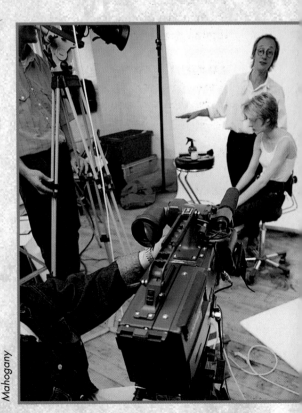

Mahogany

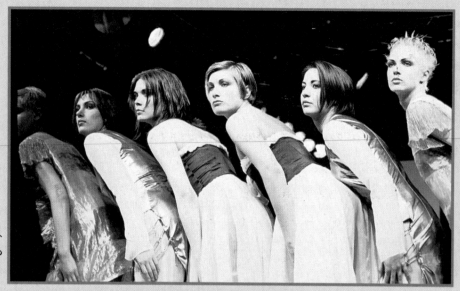

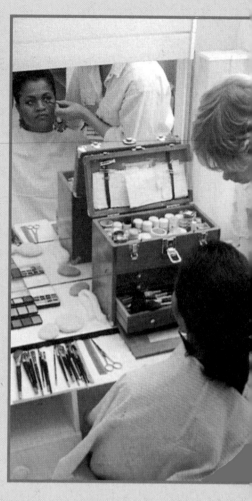

Mahogany

After qualifying in hairdressing, you may want to qualify in related skills, to open up further career routes.

● *Beauty therapists* deal with beauty treatments: they operate in hair or beauty salons.
● *Beauty specialists* offer general cosmetic and beauty treatments.
● *Manicurists, pedicurists and nail technicians* deal with the nails on the hands and feet.

● *Make-up specialists* may offer fashion, remedial or theatrical make-up.
● *Remedial make-up artists* deal with corrective make-up, disguising scars and wounds.
● *Television make-up artists* specialise in studio make-up.
● *Photographic studio specialists* deal with promotional hairstyles, and beauty photographs and advertising.

Saturday or part-time work in hairdressing

Whichever career path you choose, there are many ways of finding out more about hairdressing before committing yourself to full-time employment.

● As a beginner, you may be able to work in a salon on Saturdays or on a day-release scheme from school or college. Other schemes may allow you to work in a salon for a week or more before leaving school or college.
● Later, as a trained hairdresser, you may be able to work part-time at certain times of the week: this allows you to fit other activities into your working week.

Flexible schemes are designed to meet both your needs and your employer's needs. Approach local salons or ask your careers teacher for further information.

Start Hairdressing! is an introduction to some of the practices of hairdressing. As you can now see, there is a wide range of jobs to choose from. Remember that a broad basic training enables you to adjust and to adapt more easily later. Your success will depend a great deal on how much you enjoy what you do, and whether your actions encourage customers to return to the salon for *your* professional attention.

Answers to multiple-choice questions

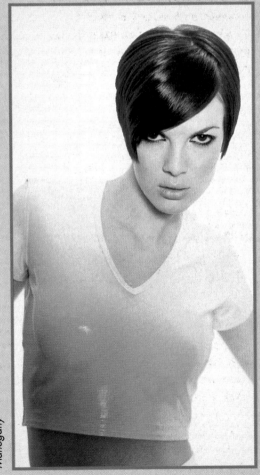

Mahogany

CHAPTER 1 1 (a) 2 (b) 3 (b)

CHAPTER 2 1 (b) 2 (b) 3 (c)

CHAPTER 3 1 (c) 2 (b) 3 (c)

CHAPTER 4 1 (c) 2 (b) 3 (a)

CHAPTER 5 1 (b) 2 (b) 3 (c)

CHAPTER 6 1 (c) 2 (a) 3 (a)

CHAPTER 7 1 (b) 2 (c) 3 (b)

Index